Do You Have Iron Overload?

There are some important new facts you should know:

- High amounts of iron can cause heart attacks and cancer and can accelerate the aging process.
- Lowering your cholesterol may not significantly prevent heart disease unless you also lower your iron level.
- The heart risks of menopause may have as much to do with increased iron levels as changes in hormones.
- Younger women do *not* need more iron in their diet.
- Over a million people in the U.S. have an inherited condition that causes them to absorb too much iron.

Iron and Your Heart is designed to translate these important new medical discoveries into simple steps you should take in order to live better and longer, with more awareness and less risk.

"But I thought iron was good for me!" you say. Well, science has marched on and left many of us in the dust. A modest amount of iron in the body *is* required for good health, but the rich diet and longer lifespan typical of modern Western society unfortunately leads to iron accumulation.

Since the original publication of this book, scientific findings about the dark side of iron have been pouring in from around the world. *The latest bombshell was a large Finnish heart disease study showing that men with elevated iron levels were at greater risk of having heart attacks.* This University of Kuopio study also showed that iron and cholesterol seemed to be working synergistically: Men with high readings of both substances were *four times as likely to have a heart attack.* People saw immediately how these findings meshed with what we knew for years about heart disease. Perhaps it is lower iron levels, not hormones, that protect women from heart disease until menopause. Perhaps it is not only the saturated fat and cholesterol in meat that is dangerous, but also the readily absorbable iron. Suddenly it appeared that we may have been poisoning ourselves all along with too much iron. Justifiably, the Finnish heart disease study made headlines throughout the U.S. and Canada.

If you are wondering whether you have iron overload and what you can do about it, this is the book for you. *Iron and Your Heart* tells you:

- How to estimate the amount of excess iron in your body with a simple ten-minute self-test you can take at home;
- What to do if your doctor says you need an iron supplement;
- How to ask your doctor for the proper iron tests;
- Whether you should take iron if you are pregnant; and
- The secrets of the optimal diet: the low-fat, low-iron lifestyle.

The news is out, from front-page stories in *The New York Times* and *The Wall Street Journal* to cover stories in *US News and World Report* and *Maclean's*: Iron, the once-beloved mineral of strength and vitality, has become the most important new risk factor in heart disease and the latest concern of all health-minded people. It is time we all stop and think about how much iron we are putting into our bodies and how to put an end to iron overload. This book shows you how.

IRON AND YOUR HEART

IRON AND YOUR HEART

The Newly Discovered Health Risks of Excess Iron—and How You Can Beat Them

Randall B. Lauffer, Ph.D.

Foreword by Baruch S. Blumberg, M.D.,

Ph.D., Nobel Laureate

St. Martin's Press   New York

The author does not directly or indirectly dispense medical advice or prescribe the use of diet, exercise, or blood donation as a form of treatment for sickness without medical approval. Nutritionists and other experts in the field of health and nutrition hold widely varying views. It is not the intent of the author to diagnose or prescribe. The intent is only to offer health information to help you cooperate with your doctor in your mutual quest for health. In the event you use this information without your doctor's approval, you are prescribing for yourself, which is your constitutional right, but the publisher and author assume no responsibility.

Library of Congress Cataloging-in-Publication Data

Lauffer, Randall Byron
    Iron and your heart / Randall B. Lauffer ; foreword by Baruch S.
Blumberg.
        p.   cm.
    ISBN 0-312-09469-8
    1. Coronary heart disease—Etiology.   2. Iron—Toxicology.
3. Iron in the body.   I. Title.
RC685.C6L37   1993
616.1′23071—dc20   93-14712
                                                                         CIP

First Paperback Edition: June 1993

10 9 8 7 6 5 4 3 2 1

Formerly titled *Iron Balance*

To Alice, for her love and encouragement.

To Sam and Ruby, for their love, everlasting optimism, and health consciousness.

Contents

Contents

List of Figures

Acknowledgments

My greatest thanks, respect, and admiration go to the hundreds of scientists whose work on iron metabolism has paved the way for a new look at this double-edged nutrient. They are, of course, too numerous to mention, but their efforts are recorded, in part, in their published works cited at the end of this book.

Special thanks go to Drs. William Crosby, Richard Stevens, Jerome Sullivan, and Gene Weinberg, the true pioneers of the new commonsense approach to dietary iron. My many conversations with them and their comments on the manuscript in its early stages were invaluable. I also thank Drs. Phil Aisen, Victor Herbert, and Jay Zweier for helpful discussions, and Drs. T. Colin Campbell and Banoo Parpia, investigators in a large nutritional study in China, for providing scientific results prior to publication.

Roberta Crawford, president of the Iron Overload Diseases Association, provided a great deal of information on her organization's efforts to increase awareness of this condition, and she was instrumental in getting me in touch with iron-overload victims and their families. Of these patients and relatives, I thank Jennifer Hyland and her mother, Louise (treasurer of the IOD Association), Hedwig Mury, wife of the late John Mury, and the others who spoke to me at length about the difficulties of getting properly diagnosed and their earnest hope that spreading the word will prevent others from suffering as they did. I also thank Dr. Margaret Krikker, president of the Hemochromatosis Research Foundation, for illuminating discussions on the forces allied against the commonsense approach to iron.

I am indebted to my own doctor, Dr. George Cohen, and his nurses for acquiescing to my puzzling demands for numerous blood tests to measure the effects of the Iron Balance Health Plan on my iron levels. The kind nurses at the Massachusetts General Hospital Blood Transfusion Service also deserve special mention for leading this cowardly novice through his first few blood donations and telling some great stories along the way.

I should also thank Drs. Tom Brady, Bruce Rosen, Bruce Jenkins, Michelle Neuder, and other fellow researchers at the Massachusetts General Hospital who patiently overlooked my occasionally harried state during the preparation of this book. Special thanks go to Dr. Leena Porkka at MGH for providing the insider's of the Finnish diet.

The book owes a great deal to the creativity and professionalism of Jared Kieling, my editor at St. Martin's Press, and Ensley Eikenburg, both of whom were a pleasure to work with. I also thank Russ Wild for additional editorial assistance.

My literary agent, John Ware, is beyond comparison. He focused my scattered energies in the early conceptual phase of the book and then shepherded me through the complex and sometimes troubling maze of the publishing industry. (I should also mention anonymously two literary agents who infuriated me enough to write the book with the following response to my early ideas: "It might make a very good magazine article, but not a book.")

Additional editorial assistance as well as plenty of love and encouragement came from my parents, Sam and Ruby Lauffer, whose lifelong curiosity about diet and health has stimulated my own. My mother-in-law, Janine Vincent, contributed the same; she is one of my best critics, but only in the literary sense.

Finally, my utmost thanks go to my wife, Alice, whose love, patience, encouragement, and "in-house" editing skills are what actually made the book a reality.

Foreword

The evaluation of the effects of nutrition on health is of great interest to many; there is an intuitive belief that the food which we volitionally introduce into our own bodies must have a great influence on health, disease, and general well-being. In addition, nutrition is a factor that, within limits, many people can control themselves and about which they have to make their own decisions. There is enormous interest in food: in growing it, preparing it, eating it, and the social and personal ceremonies surrounding it. That we are what we eat may or may not be true, but there are many who believe that it is.

Despite this great concern, it is difficult to accurately evaluate the effects of food on disease. The input variables in the equation—the fats, carbohydrates, proteins, vitamins, minerals, total calories, and so on—are very large, and the possible outcome variables, including heart disease, various kinds of cancer, and a host of other diseases, are also numerous. The statistical methods available to evaluate such variables are inadequate and in any case would require studies of vast numbers of subjects at enormous expense. Furthermore, only a few variables can be considered in any study, and sometimes what are subsequently found to be essential variables have not been included in the original study design. As a consequence, the conclusions of one study may be upset by a subsequent one, to the distress of the consumers and often the producers and processors of the food in question. Even more often, because of the difficulty of executing enormous control studies, those that are done, or have been done in the past when the methods of clinical and epidemiological evaluation were less developed, are inadequate and their conclusions invalid.

It is not surprising that there is great reliance on anecdotal information; for example, the advice that parents give their children endlessly as they are growing and maturing—in fact, in many cases, even beyond that time. There is now a focus as well on specialized diets to whose value their practitioners provide convincing testimony. There is hardly any field of medicine and health care in which more weight is given to personal and scientifically untested opinion.

Despite these caveats, valid comparisons of diet constituents have been done and, particularly in recent years, they are based on sound and well-conceived study plans. Many of these have been presented by Dr. Randall B. Lauffer in this book on iron and health.

There is a widespread belief that if a little of something is good, then a lot is better. The belief arises from what might be called a linear view of biology. For example, it is known that a small amount of vitamin C can prevent and cure the horrible consequences of scurvy, and vitamin B those of beri-beri. The inference has then been made that an increased amount of these constituents may not only repair any damage due to the deficiency, but be valuable in a whole manner of other biological mechanisms in people who are not suffering from disease. This view can often be supported by directed experiments with accompanying biological and chemical arguments to explain the postulated outcome. Despite this, for many biological systems, an insufficient amount of a substance may be detrimental, but also, a large amount beyond a certain optimal amount may also be detrimental.

This appears to be the case for iron, and Dr. Lauffer has assembled a variety of data to support this contention. Iron is valuable for the treatment of iron-deficiency anemia, a disease common in many countries in which nutrition is poor, but also in relatively wealthy countries in persons whose nutritional habits are poor, or during certain periods of life when iron demands are increased. However, in most advanced societies, this form of anemia is not widespread. It is probably best treated by administering iron to those who require it and not to the entire population by the supplementation of widely used foodstuffs or the common prescription of iron tablets to those who do not specifically require them. Moreover, there is a growing body of evidence that excess iron intake may be unwise and even dangerous to many in the society who are now receiving supplementary iron.

Over the years, numerous experimental studies showed that, in animals and in humans, greater amounts of available iron increase the possibility of infection and the development of cancer and other forms of illness. These phenomena have been studied and discussed extensively by Dr. Eugene Weinberg at Indiana University.

The interest in iron in my own laboratory at the Fox Chase Cancer Center in Philadelphia started after evidence began to accumulate that hepatitis B virus, in which we had been interested for many years, was involved with the cause of primary cancer of the liver, a very serious and common disease in many parts of Asia, Africa, and South America and to a lesser extent elsewhere. We were often asked if there were any effects attributable to food and were urged by the funding agencies to investigate the effect of nutrition on this form of cancer. We decided to study iron because of our prior interests in it and the relative ease of conducting clinical and epidemiologic studies. Only small amounts of blood were necessary for many of the measurements and, at least initially, detailed nutritional surveys were not essential.

From our first investigations we inferred that increased iron stores in the cells infected with hepatitis B virus increased the replication (that is, the reproduction) of the virus. Later, we learned that increased iron stores were associated with a greater likelihood that a person already infected with hepatitis virus would develop primary cancer of the liver.

Dr. Richard Stevens, at that time in my laboratory, embarked on a series of epidemiological studies employing a somewhat curious use of time. We had over the years accumulated blood and other biological specimens from populations that had been studied for biochemical and immunological variation, and to understand the epidemiology of hepatitis B virus. These sera had been stored (in many cases for twenty years or more), and we were able to use them for what have been called "historic prospective" epidemiologic studies. They are "historic" in that the blood samples have been preserved for a relatively long time and "prospective" in that they look forward from the blood samples' past into the subjects' future, that is, the present. The first such study was done on populations living in the Solomon

Islands who had been the subjects of an intensive health survey combined with treatment and prevention programs conducted by the late Alfred Damon in the 1960s and early 1970s. These included the collection of blood specimens. Some twenty years after the first collections, a repeat visit to the islands established who was alive or dead.

We wanted to test the hypothesis that increased body stores of iron were associated with decreased survival. We selected the stored sera from those who died and compared them to a control group of people who had survived. We predicted that survival would be associated with lower body iron stores as estimated by the blood levels of certain proteins. The analysis of the data confirmed these predictions. Following this and some of the subsequent studies, we recommended that additional attempts to test this hypothesis should be made with the possibility that in due course the practices of iron supplementation and treatment would be altered.

A powerful tool that can be used in epidemiologic studies is the technique of independent evidence. Epidemiologic studies usually involve a large number of variables, some known and even more unknown. It is very difficult to duplicate exactly an original study for which validation is sought. It is more feasible and powerful to design a different study to test the same hypothesis. These secondary validating studies will often involve different populations, times, and circumstances; in fact, a new set of variables. If the hypothesis is confirmed in the secondary studies, powerful support is given to the hypothesis in that the investigator can assert that even with a different set of variables the hypothesis prevails. Conversely, while an argument can often be raised to refute one set of arguments, the same objection is unlikely to refute the body of evidence produced by the subsequent studies.

To that end, additional studies were done by Dr. Stevens and his colleagues and other investigators. In one of these, conducted in Taiwan, it was shown that increased iron stores were associated with the development of primary cancer of the liver and other cancers. In subsequent studies in Taiwan, the United States, and elsewhere, the hypothesis that increased body iron stores are associated with increased risk for some, but not all, cancers was supported. One study conducted in Europe was reported to have refuted the association, but the full details of this investigation were not available. In addition a series of observations (many by Dr. Hei-won Hann and her associates at the Fox Chase Cancer Center) were made on laboratory animals whose iron intake was varied, and these also gave additional independent support to the concept.

These observations on the general population have been made even more acute with the realization that the inherited disease hemochromatosis, in which there is excessive accumulation of iron, is much more common than previously estimated. There is also the possibility that individuals with the mild form of the disease, who make up a sizable fraction of the population, might be at increased risk if they ingest large amounts of iron.

Often, an accumulation of a large body of evidence is required before the public is motivated to change health practices. For example, even though significant evidence that cigarette smoking was detrimental began to accumulate in the 1950s, it wasn't until recently that there were changes in public health practice. An increased awareness of the possible hazards of increased iron intake may now be developing, and this could stimulate additional research and ultimately public action. A possible example of this is a meeting held in April 1991 by the Department of Medical Nutrition and other departments of the Karolinska Hospital in Stockholm to discuss some of the detrimental effects of long-term overuse of iron. Sweden, like America, has an active program for the iron enrichment of flour, and iron supplements are widely used by the general population. There was some media attention focused on the meeting, and it's possible that in the future this may lead to further action by the public health authorities.

Dr. Lauffer's *Iron Balance*, directed to a general audience, can also affect perceptions on this problem. It presents the data in an easily accessible style. The recommendations given are by no means radical. They suggest stopping the use of iron supplements unless there is some clear indication that they are required. The further recommendation that, within medically acceptable limits, iron levels could be reduced by occasional blood donation also has merit even though it will take some time before the actual effects on health can be determined directly. (A recent study from Sweden is consistent with a beneficial effect but must be confirmed by additional studies.) If public action is in due course taken based on the recommendations of the earlier researches and *Iron Balance*, it might have the secondary effect of questioning the use of other food supplements and initiating additional research on their long-term effects.

—Baruch S. Blumberg, M.D., Ph.D.
  Fox Chase Distinguished Scientist, Fox Chase Cancer Center, Philadelphia
  Master, Balliol College, Oxford University
  Recipient of the 1976 Nobel Prize in Physiology or Medicine

Introduction:
A Message to Change Your Mind

Among nutrients, iron is, I think, one of the least understood. Despite enormous evidence to the contrary, the public and most nutritionists continue to view iron in far too rosy a light. Iron is thought of as the nutrient of strength, the secret ingredient in Popeye's spinach. Its dark side, which threatens the health of millions of Americans, is seldom discussed.

Here are some common myths about iron that you may have heard:

- Iron deficiency is the number-one nutritional problem in the U.S.
- Most women need more iron than they are getting from their diet.
- People over fifty don't get enough iron.
- You need meat in your diet to get enough iron.
- Liver, a good source of iron, is one of the most nutritious and healthy meats.
- Iron overload, wherein the body contains too much iron, is an extremely rare condition.

As you will read in the pages that follow, *these reasonable-sounding ideas are all completely false!* Recent scientific findings have refuted many of these long-held beliefs; the others we have simply clung to despite information to the contrary, which we have had for some time.

How has this occurred? We have been misled by drug companies pushing iron supplements. We have been misled by nutritionists who all too often focused on nutritional deficiencies, not nutritional excesses. And we have been misled by our own

1

old-fashioned, fanciful ideas about iron, the magical nutrient of strength.

The main problem with iron is not with too little but with too much. In iron, nature has harnessed some powerful chemical potential, mostly to good, even astounding, use. But there are a few glitches in the way our bodies handle this powerful substance. Over time, we absorb too much iron from our rich diet. It is then more likely to take its chemical potential into the wrong place at the wrong time, unleashing damage to vital structures within our cells.

Nature has more or less done a halfway job in tackling these problems: since reproduction, not longevity, is the ultimate goal of life, nature has made sure that iron's nasty side is held in check during the early fertile years. But aging is, unfortunately, accompanied by some not-so-graceful chemistry. Recent research findings have indicated that nature's flimsy control over iron and other active substances may contribute to cancer, heart disease, and several other common degenerative diseases of our day.

The good news is that you can do something about it. I estimate that roughly half of the population, especially adult men and postmenopausal women, are iron-overloaded to some extent and should reduce their iron levels. The goal is Iron Balance, by which I mean the state in which iron stores in the body are sufficient but not excessive, and the absorption of iron from the diet balances daily losses. This book tells you how to get there. Along with a proper diet and plenty of exercise, Iron Balance can bring you one step closer to the fabled fountain of youth.

To your health!

Part 1

IRON: FACT AND FICTION

1

Our One-Sided View of Iron

What pops into your mind when you think of iron? Fabulous steel skyscrapers? The iron bars that separate convicted murderers from the rest of us? Something you use at home to flatten the wrinkles in clothes into oblivion? Grandma's skillet?

Now think of iron, the nutrient. Now and then you see it listed in the nutritional tables on food packaging. You may be a little disappointed when you see that a single serving of Oreos or Doritos gives you "less than 2% of the Recommended Daily Allowance" of iron. But you always feel a little better in the morning when you read that your breakfast cereal provides 25 percent and in some cases 100 percent of the RDA for iron. You may remember your mother telling you to finish your plate of liver so that you could get enough iron to grow up big and strong. It is nice, you think, to live in a modern age where we don't need to eat liver anymore. You head out for a busy day, letting that iron work its special magic.

From Popeye the Sailor Man to Geritol, the relief for "iron-poor blood," many elements in our culture have influenced our positive view of iron as a nutrient. Iron has connotations of strength, vitality, and even sexual potency. We cannot get enough of the stuff.

Now think of cholesterol. A few images of cheesecake or thick, juicy steaks might flash through your mind, inevitably followed by the thought of clogged arteries and heart attacks. *It* is all bad, or at least tinged with guilt. "Cholesterol-free" is the only thing that sounds good about cholesterol.

Why should iron's reputation be so good and cholesterol's so bad? In a general sense, they have a lot in common. Both are substances required for our good health. Take all the cholesterol out of your body and the very framework of cellular structure, your cell walls, would weaken and disintegrate. Your tissues would no longer be able to synthesize a cascade of cholesterol by-products that communicate important messages throughout your body. Similarly, with no iron, you would lack the ability to transport and utilize that life-giving gas, oxygen. Even the very essence of life, DNA, the genetic material in our chromosomes, would no longer be synthesized; new cell growth would halt.

But iron, as well as cholesterol, has a flip side. Cholesterol's is all too familiar and understandable. The Western world loves the fatty foods that give rise to high cholesterol levels. No more need be said. The dark side of iron, on the other hand, is less familiar. We are generally unaware that this dissolved metal can act like an atomic cannonball, wreaking havoc in our tissues when it is present in excess or is simply in the wrong place at the wrong time. Few of us—and, unfortunately, few doctors—know this side of iron.

It is almost as if iron has had an excellent public relations consultant throughout history. Iron has been with us since the Iron Age, whereas cholesterol, relatively speaking, was discovered only yesterday. We can associate nutritional iron with the characteristics of the glimmering skyscrapers and hard tools made of metallic iron: strength, durability, perhaps even immortality. But what is cholesterol? A waxy, white, amorphous substance with a bad reputation.

Let us take a look at how iron became an important part of our culture, and how this has influenced our view of the metal in health and nutrition.

The Iron Age

The beginning of the story is, naturally, the Iron Age. In the transitions from the Stone Age to the Bronze Age to the Iron Age, the hardness and durability of armaments and tools were steadily improved. These developments were accompanied by drastic changes in ancient civilizations.

The most important event associated with the discovery of iron is the fall of the creative and powerful ancient Egyptian civilization. Egypt had garnered a great deal of its power from its control of the large copper deposits in the Sinai Peninsula. Copper, the main ingredient in bronze, gave the Egyptians tremendous advantages over other civilizations. However, by the thirteenth century B.C., other societies developed the technology to utilize iron in tools and weapons. Iron, in addition to its greater hardness, had the important advantage of being found in much larger quantities in many more places than copper. This resulted in larger, more powerfully equipped armies. The Egyptian army was no match for these iron armies from the north and, for the nearly three thousand years that followed, Egypt was no longer an independent country.

As a result, iron has earned a respectable place in history. The great English historian Edward Gibbon wrote in 1776, "It has been observed . . . that the command of iron soon gives a nation the command of gold."[1] Another important reference to iron is in the first encyclopedia, the massive *The Historie of the World*, written in the first century A.D. by Gaius Plinius Secundus, known to friends as Pliny the Elder. Here is a quotation from an Old English translation dating back to 1601:[2]

> It remaineth now to discourse of . . . yron, a mettal which wee may well say is both the best and the worst . . . in the world: For with the help of yron we breake up and ear the ground, we plant and plot our groves, we set our hort-yards . . . by means of yron and steele we build houses, hew quarries . . . yea and in one word, we use it to all other necessarie uses of this life. Contrariwise, the same yron serveth for warres, murders, and robberies . . . this I take

to bee the wickedest invention that ever was devised by the
head of man. . . .

As you will see, this combination of constructive and destructive
elements applies equally well to the role iron plays in human
health and nutrition.

Early Prescriptions for the "Metal of Heaven"

In their quest for improved health, ancient peoples ingested and
applied to their bodies a wide variety of herbs and potions containing potentially toxic chemicals. They would try anything
their "medicine man" dreamed up. Modern medicine had thousands of years of experience with human guinea pigs from which
to select promising treatments. Many of these treatments have
turned out to make sense in the light of modern science, but
others were only fanciful.

Since iron was thought of as the "metal of heaven"—some
scholars think this was because of the high iron content found
in meteorites that had fallen from the sky—it was only a matter
of time before someone tried it as a medicine. The first "prescription" for iron can be found in the oldest recorded document,
the Egyptian medicine book *Ebers Papyrus*, which dates back to
about 1500 B.C.[3] It is, oddly enough, a prescription for a potion—
and some magic words—to treat baldness:

> "O shining One, thou who hoverest above!
> O Xare! O disc of the sun!
> O protector of the divine Neb-Apt!"
> to be spoken over
> Iron
> Red lead
> Onions
> Alabaster
> Honey
> make into one and give against.

In the Greco-Roman period, iron was regarded as a gift of the god of war, known to the Greeks as Ares and to the Romans as Mars. Iron was often applied directly to battle wounds, since it was believed that the contact with the original weapon would aid healing.[3]

The first use of orally administered iron to obtain strength appears to be in Greek mythology. Legend has it that Jason and his Argonauts would sharpen their iron swords, letting the filings drop into acidic red wine. It was supposed to be the savage power of the weapon that gave the wine its empowering force. But we now know that some of the iron would dissolve in the acidic wine, providing, at most, an iron supplement.[4]

Another Greek legend purported that a similar potion cured the mythical Prince Iphylus of impotence. The prince was unable to beget a child and consulted his local medicine man. Using a method that would delight Freudians, the doctor had the prince talk about his childhood. It turned out that the prince had suffered a severe emotional blow as a child. He had watched his father perform the gelding of a lamb and was frightened by the blood-covered knife. The knife remained, both in the prince's mind and at the site of the operation, for his father had driven the bloody knife into a nearby oak tree. Doctors today guess that in later years the prince understandably would be suffering from castration anxiety. The prince's medicine man may have had a different term for it, but his recommended treatment seemed right on the mark: the prince must confront his fears by chopping down the oak tree, recovering the knife, and preparing a potion of wine mixed with filings from the rusty knife. The prince was cured, his manhood restored, and the royal lineage was maintained. Though it was only indirectly responsible for the "cure" in this case, iron and its magical effects had nevertheless found their way into the folklore of the time.[3]

Curing Green Virgins With Iron

We now know that the only justified medical use of iron is in the treatment of true iron deficiency. A sustained lack of iron leads to anemia, a reduced capacity of the blood to carry oxygen, which makes its victims pale and listless. For this condition, iron is indeed a miracle drug. The story behind the discovery of iron as a treatment for anemia is rich with amusing misdiagnoses and cures.

For thousands of years, iron-deficiency anemia was common among young girls after the onset of puberty. These girls failed to get enough iron to keep up with the dual demands of growth and iron loss through menstruation. Their pale faces, for unknown reasons, often had a green tint, leading to the popular term "greensickness" and the medical term *chlorosis* (from the Greek word for *green*). Writers from Hippocrates to Shakespeare mentioned this curious disease, and several artists, particularly seventeenth-century Dutch artists, captured the image of chlorotic women in oil paintings.[5]

The first medical description of chlorosis was by the Dutch physician Johannes Lange. In 1554, Lange wrote to a friend who had a sick daughter, surprised that no other doctor had diagnosed her properly:[6]

> You complain to me . . . that your eldest daughter, Anna, is now marriageable, and has many eligible suitors, all of whom you are obliged to dismiss on account of her ill-health, the cause of which no doctor can discover. . . . Wherefore you entreat me by our ancient friendship to give an opinion on her case, with advice as to marriage, and you send me an excellent account of her symptoms. Her face which last year showed rosy cheeks and lips, has become pale and bloodless, her heart palpitates at every moment, and the pulse is visible in the temporal arteries; she loses her breath when dancing or going upstairs, she dislikes her food, especially meat, and her legs swell towards the ankles. I marvel that your physicians have not diagnosed the case from such typical symptoms. It is the affection, which the women of Brabant call the "white fever," or love sickness, for lovers are always pale. . . .

It was quite common to regard this condition as a "love sickness" because it seemed frequently to affect young, unmarried women, particularly those thought to have suffered unrequited love. (One of the famous Dutch paintings by Gerrit Dou was actually entitled *Mal d'Amour,* or "Love Sickness.") The wistful mood of these poor damsels is best captured in Shakespeare's description of Viola in *Twelfth Night:*[3]

> She never told her love
> But let concealment, like a worm in the bud
> Feed upon her damask cheek; she pined in thought
> And, with a green and yellow melancholy
> She sat, like patience on a monument.

What was the cure in those days? Marriage was often thought to be the best medicine. Johannes Lange, the first to identify "the sickness of virgins," offered this commonsense advice in the letter referred to earlier: "I therefore say, I instruct, virgins afflicted with this disease, that as soon as possible they live with men & copulate."[7]

Why were these particular women so iron-deficient? Modern-day nutrition sleuths have conjectured that these girls were not getting enough meat, the best source of iron. For example, the squeamish Victorians actually thought that spicy dishes and meats aroused sexual appetites, and these dishes were often withheld from young girls to keep their yearnings at bay. This practice was especially popular in cities and towns. Country girls, on the other hand, apparently had a more natural, balanced diet and, according to some medical historians, had less of a problem with chlorosis. Even before the Victorian age, "natural girls" from the country were thought to have some special charm, as expressed in this passage from Izaak Walton's *The Compleat Angler* (1653):[3]

> I married a wife of late,
> The more's my unhappy fate:
> I married her for love
> As my fancy did me move,
> And not for a worldly estate.
> But oh! the green-sickness
> Soon changed her likeness;
> And all her beauty did fail.

> But 'tis not so
> With those that go
> Thro' frost and snow
> As all men know
> And carry the milking pail.

Eventually certain folk remedies, including iron filings dissolved in wine, were identified as more effective treatments for chlorosis than marriage or certain other activities. These, of course, actually solved the iron-deficiency problem, though physicians at that time had no idea why the treatments were working. One of the more interesting customs passed on from mother to daughter involved sticking a number of nails into an apple, removing them after a few hours, and eating the apple.[4] We now can understand that trace amounts of iron must have dissolved into the apple, and it was this that brought color back into the cheeks.

The man credited with discovering iron as a specific remedy for chlorosis was Thomas Sydenham of London. In the late 1600s, he wrote a classic description of the effects of a "steel tonic":[3]

> I comfort the blood and the spirits belonging to it by giving [iron] thirty days running. . . . The pulse gains strength and frequency, the surface warmth, the face (no longer pale and deathlike) a fresh ruddy color. . . .
>
> Next to steel in substance, I prefer a syrup. This is made by steeping iron or steel filings in cold Rhenish wine. When the wine is sufficiently impregnated, strain the liquor; add sugar; and boil to the consistency of syrup.

As science marched on, it was discovered that iron is an important constituent of blood. When most of the iron in blood was found to be part of the oxygen-carrying protein molecule called *hemoglobin*, the treatment of anemia with supplemental iron finally made complete sense. When the body is deficient in iron, the dark red hemoglobin molecules cannot be synthesized; lower hemoglobin levels in the blood lead to poor oxygen delivery and the pale cheeks of anemia.

Though it took a great deal of convincing, doctors finally agreed that chlorosis was caused by iron deficiency. However, many still thought it was a female nervous disorder and that iron was an effective placebo. Persuasive evidence was offered in 1893 by Ralph Stockman, a lecturer at the School of Medicine in Edinburgh, Scotland. He showed clearly that the hemoglobin levels in chlorotic women were raised after iron treatment. He also performed one of the first nutritional analyses focused on iron: he found that his own diet provided approximately 9 milligrams of iron per day; that of a normal, healthy young woman, 8 milligrams per day; and that of two chlorotic girls, 1.3–3.4 milligrams per day. The sick girls were obviously not getting enough iron to replace their average daily losses.[3]

Soon after these discoveries, simple iron supplements became available for medicinal purposes. In addition, iron-deficiency anemia could be detected earlier by measuring hemoglobin levels in blood. These factors combined to wipe "greensickness" off the medical map.[8]

Lingering Notions

Today a much milder form of iron-deficiency anemia can occur in developed countries, though it is not as common as many people think. As you will learn in Part 2, the prevalence of anemia in America has been grossly exaggerated by certain factors within our medical, industrial, and governmental organizations. I cannot help but think that cultural notions may have had something to do with this.

While the legends of Prince Iphylus and the warrior Jason are buried today, the notion that iron gives you strength lives on. Consider Popeye the Sailor Man, for instance. He is by far the most popular of "nutritional heroes" in the twentieth century. The bulky-armed sailor first appeared in Elzie Segar's comic strip "Thimble Theatre" in 1929 and soon stole the show. In defending his beloved Olive Oyl from arch rival Bluto, he would gulp down a can of spinach to lend him strength, singing "I'm strong to the finish 'cause I eats my spinach." There was even a statue of

Popeye in the central square of Crystal City, Texas, an important spinach-growing center. People came to believe that it was the iron in the spinach that gave him stamina, and Popeye and iron were forever linked in many people's minds. (Ironically, we now know that the iron in spinach is not well absorbed during digestion.)

One company, the original makers of the modern-day iron potion, Geritol, capitalized on this prevailing myth that iron will give you strength and, through deceptive advertising, persuaded millions of people to take excess supplements of this potentially dangerous mineral. Geritol, the ads said, "has twice the iron in a pound of calf's liver" and will make you "feel strong fast." In short, Geritol is supposed to give you "iron power." Chapter 3 reveals the truth behind this scam and the company's long battle with the Federal Trade Commission.

A New Wind Blows

More than ever we need to put our cultural influences behind us and get the facts about iron. While the symbolism of iron as a magical substance is great for getting kids to eat their spinach, it has no place in our modern world, where double-edged nutrients are a fact of life and the key word is *balance*. Just as metallic iron can be molded into a harmless horseshoe or a fierce sword, the potential of iron to perform unique and powerful chemical reactions can turn against us. This Jekyll-to-Hyde transformation of iron is quite common and may play a role in some of our most deadly ailments, such as heart disease and cancer.

Cold Iron: The Master of Them All

If you want more fitting symbolism for iron, consider the Rudyard Kipling story "Cold Iron" in his book *Rewards and Fairies*. The story tells of how the King and Queen of Fairyland adopt a human baby, the orphan son of a slave woman. They teach the boy magic with the intent that he become the Prince of Fairyland. But there is a special condition of his adoption: they must prohibit the boy from touching "Cold Iron" until he reaches manhood. When he does, the object containing the iron will determine his future.

One day the King and Queen are watching the prince play, and he bends over to pick up something on the ground. Immediately they know it is "Cold Iron" and anxiously wait to see what the future will hold. Is it an iron scepter crowned with jewels? Then he may become king! Is it a magnificent sword? That would mean he may become a knight! Or maybe it is a book of learning, bound with iron clasps.

In the distance the parents see the boy fastening something around his neck: alas, it is an iron slave ring. Our narrator tells us that unfortunately the boy must now return to the common folk:

> Never will he be his own master, nor yet ever any man's. He will get half he gives, and give twice what he gets, till his life's last breath; and if he lays aside his load before he draws that last breath, all his work will go for naught.
>
> [Common folk] are born on the near side of Cold Iron— there's iron in every man's house, isn't there? They handle Cold Iron every day of their lives, and their fortune's made or spoilt by Cold Iron in some shape or other. That's how it goes with Flesh and Blood, and one can't prevent it.

There are often many layers of meaning within a Kipling story, and I don't think he would mind if we add one of our own to this poignant tale. As you will see in the following chapters, iron has enslaved the health of us common folk. We let it creep into our bodies, and we slowly rust away, so to speak. Our tissues simply cannot stand too much iron: too many things can go wrong. "That's how it goes with Flesh and Blood."

So, think not of Popeye and superhuman strength when you think of iron. Remember the slave ring and these words from the poem that follows Kipling's story:

"Gold is for the mistress—silver for the maid—
Copper for the craftsman cunning at his trade."
"Good!" said the Baron, sitting in his hall,
"But Iron—Cold Iron—is master of them all."

—"Cold Iron," Rudyard Kipling

2

Iron in Your Body: Freeways and Dead Ends

Iron is required for life on this planet. If all the iron on the globe were sucked off instantaneously, all life would cease in minutes, if not seconds. Animals like us would suffer asphyxiation, and plants and bacteria would no longer be able to grow or derive energy from food. All of us, from the lowly *Escherichia coli* bacteria to man, are hooked on iron.

Iron is indeed a magical element, as ancient civilizations once believed. It can perform a wide variety of unique and marvelous chemical feats. One of the most important functions of iron in animals is the transport of oxygen in the blood. Iron is also required for the burning of "fuel"—food and body fat—and the creation of new cells to replace old ones. These, along with other crucial chemical reactions assisted by iron, make it critical for all organisms to efficiently store away excess iron in case a shortage arises. Humans are extremely good at this.

But alas, iron accumulation and its chemical power can, in certain circumstances, backfire on us, punching holes in our cell walls and disrupting our chromosomes. These tiny atom-sized cannonballs, which can be "melted down" and made into useful substances, can at the same time be destructive little wrecking balls.

Iron and Your Red Blood Cells

Let's begin this good-news-bad-news story with iron's role in the transport of oxygen, that life-giving gas. Of the teaspoon or so of iron in the human body (about two to five grams), 60 to 75 percent of it is present in the form of hemoglobin, a vital component of our highly evolved circulatory system. This mass transit system for oxygen is one of the important features that separate us from lower organisms.

An incredibly complex freeway system of arteries, capillaries, and veins is laid throughout your body; over ten billion capillaries carve intricate paths through your tissues. From the microscopic point of view, the circulatory freeway is dominated by massive red-blood-cell "buses." It is rush hour all the time: there are over twenty-five trillion of these buses being pushed and shoved through your blood vessels by the pumping actions of the heart. Placed end to end, the red blood cells from one human being would encircle the globe six times, or almost stretch to the moon. But in reality they are packed into five quarts of blood occupying about 40 percent of its volume.

The red blood cells are specifically designed for the important function of picking up oxygen in the lungs and releasing it in tissues; they also aid in the transport of the waste product, carbon dioxide, back to the lungs for exhalation. Each cell is filled to the limit with about 300 million molecules of hemoglobin, the iron-containing substance that acts as a "seat" for oxygen on the bus. The presence of hemoglobin allows our blood to carry seventy times more oxygen than could be dissolved in water alone; without it we would be sluggish and inefficient creatures at best.

Iron in Your Body Is Handled With Kid Gloves

Despite the care that goes into the assembly of red blood cells, each of them only holds up for about 120 days. You might say that they run up some pretty high numbers on the odometer, having gone through the entire circulatory system over 170,000 times. During that time a cell is squashed into a variety of shapes as it is pushed through tight capillaries. Its coat also becomes tarnished. Specialized scavenger cells in the liver, spleen, and bone marrow, collectively called the *reticuloendothelial system*, take up the old red blood cells and melt them down into iron, protein, and fat. It is recycling at its best.

Your body goes to great lengths to recycle, transport, and store all the iron released from old, broken-down red blood cells. Iron is treated almost as if it were gold. Specialized proteins have evolved to take care of these tasks.

One of these proteins, ferritin, stores excess iron inside cells. (The prefix *ferri-* derives from *ferrum*, the Latin word for iron.) These ferritin "storage bins" exist in every type of cell, guarding against iron deficiency that might arise because of bleeding or dietary inadequacy.

Ferritin is a huge spherical protein, a molecular version of Buckminster Fuller's geodesic dome. Inside the vast interior of a ferritin molecule, iron atoms can stick to the protein walls, layering on top of one another. Although there is room for up to 4500 iron atoms, there is usually a maximum of about 2000 stored inside. The chemical form of the iron is similar to that of rust, and as it sits inside the dome, it cannot do us much harm. Under some conditions, however, the iron can be released, either through tiny portholes in the protein wall or through the destruction of the entire molecule. You might say that the iron atoms are safely stored away; but as with cannonballs stored next to a cannon, their destructive power can still be unleashed.

A second important protein that evolved to transport iron in the blood is named, appropriately enough, *transferrin*. This protein is a sort of molecular wheelbarrow, with room for only two iron atoms. The empty wheelbarrow picks up iron from decomposed red blood cells or absorbed foods and delivers it to other cells that need it.

By virtue of the very efficient recycling of hemoglobin iron, our daily requirement for iron from food is really quite small. We do lose iron, about one milligram per day, in the form of sweat and urine, as well as in cells that naturally slough off from the intestinal wall, hair, skin, and nails. Premenopausal women must also replace an additional .6 milligram of iron per day (calculated over the month), which is lost in menstruation. This means that absorbing only about 1–1.6 milligrams per day of iron from food, equivalent to the total amount of iron in half a McDonald's hamburger or a small bowl of Kellogg's cornflakes, will prevent us from getting anemic.[1-4]

If we do become truly iron deficient, our bodies have an efficient way of dealing with the problem: the absorption of iron from food in the intestine increases considerably to alleviate the deficiency. Unless the average daily loss of iron is very large, from heavily bleeding tissue, for example, this protective mechanism works well. Most menstruating women are not iron deficient because this absorption mechanism performs effectively. In addition, if they still need more iron, they can draw on their reserves in ferritin "storage bins."

Iron Is Trapped Inside Your Body

What about excess iron? Can our bodies excrete it? The answer is, surprisingly, *no*. In stark contrast to the elegant system evolved to get iron *into* the body and to store it, we have no effective and regulated way to rid ourselves of excess iron. This is even more surprising in light of the way our bodies carefully regulate other dissolved metals, such as potassium.

In the early days of the twentieth century, most investigators assumed that, since the feces contain substantial amounts of iron, the intestines must excrete it. But this iron comes, in fact, mostly from the diet. The scientific world was set straight on this issue in 1937 by the work of Drs. Robert McCance and Elsie Widdowson of King's College Hospital in London. Here is how Dr. Widdowson described their discovery years later:[5]

> It all started with a patient, Mrs. Harris, who was suffering from polycythemia rubra vera. This disease is characterized by far too many red blood cells, and consequently very sticky blood. One treatment was to give a drug called phenylhydrazine. This drug causes breakdown of the red cells and when this happens the iron in the hemoglobin in

the red cells is set free inside the body. We reckoned that Mrs. Harris had about twice as much iron in her body as a normal person, ten grams instead of five grams. We measured the amount of iron in Mrs. Harris' food and drink, and in urine and feces while she was having the drug. We fully expected Mrs. Harris to excrete far more iron than she took in in her food as the drug took effect, but to our astonishment almost all the five grams or so of iron from the broken down red cells stayed inside her body and virtually none was excreted.

We then looked carefully at the literature on the absorption and excretion of iron and we came to the conclusion that practically no iron is excreted either by the intestine or by the kidneys, and that the amount of iron in the body is maintained by controlled absorption.

We put this idea to the test by injecting intravenously into ourselves and our friends measured amounts of an iron salt every day for 14 days, and following our intakes and excretions of iron while we were doing so. Again we found that very little of the iron injected was excreted. So our hypothesis seemed to be correct, and it has been proved to be so many times since.

As mentioned in the passage above, we do have a somewhat naturally regulated, but unfortunately inefficient, mechanism that is supposed to prevent iron overload: "controlled absorption." As the body's iron stores increase, the absorption of iron by the intestinal cells decreases. Some scientists, particularly those most concerned about iron deficiency rather than iron excess, have regarded this "absorption block" mechanism as a natural and very effective protection against iron overload: if the body does not need any more iron, the intestines simply do not absorb it. But there is an abundance of evidence that this mechanism is only partially effective: while absorption rates do decrease with more body iron, the metal still gets into the body and continuously builds up.[6-8] While the iron may not be getting into the front door, it might be sneaking in through the back. You might say that we have a very low-tech protective factor at best.

The Accumulation of Iron As We Age

One of the largest and most important studies showing that humans are iron accumulators is a 1976 paper in the journal *Blood*.[9] Drs. James Cook, Clement Finch, and Nathan Smith of the University of Washington and the University of Kansas collected and analyzed blood samples in over 1500 people living in Washington State. They employed what was then a relatively new analysis, the serum ferritin measurement, that indirectly gauges the amount of iron stored away in the tissues. You will recall that ferritin is the "storage bin" for iron that is present in all cells. For unknown reasons, some freshly synthesized ferritin with little or no iron inside leaks out of certain cells and is found floating around in the blood. The level of serum ferritin is, except in certain disease states, controlled by the level of iron stored in cells through a well-defined and well-regulated mechanism: the more iron present, the more storage bins produced and found in the blood. The simplest assumption is that one unit (a "unit" is one microgram per liter of blood serum, or one nanogram per milliliter) of serum ferritin corresponds to roughly 10 milligrams of stored iron.

The Washington State study found that serum ferritin levels, and thus iron stores, increase as we age. Figure 2-1 shows the average amount of stored iron for men and women, calculated using the simple assumption above. Both male and female youths have only moderate iron stores, since the iron demands of growth are considerable. But at around age twenty, look what happens to the iron stores in men: they jump from around 200–300 milligrams to over 800 milligrams. After that, men appear to continue to accumulate iron as they age. An overall accumulation rate for men throughout their lifetime is about twenty milligrams per year.

Women are generally protected from this burden of iron during the childbearing years, and they have moderate but adequate stores of around 200–300 milligrams. However, at menopause, when menstruation, their extra iron-loss mechanism, ceases to operate, they begin to accumulate iron rapidly, approaching the values in men (600–800 milligrams). The best way to look at the male-female difference in iron accumulation is to consider that

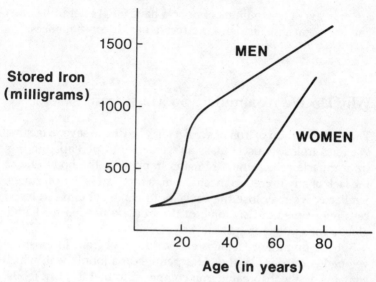

Figure 2-1. Iron accumulation with aging. This plot shows the degree to which excess iron accumulates as we age. The results are based on a large study of serum ferritin levels in Americans (Cook, J. D.; Finch, C. A.; Smith, N. J. *Blood* 48 [1976]: 449–455). After adolescence, the average iron stores in men build up rapidly and appear to continue to rise throughout their lifetime. This process is delayed some twenty to thirty years in women because of the regular iron loss due to menstruation, but once menopause is reached (at roughly age forty-five to fifty-five), women begin to accumulate iron rapidly.

menstruation in women generally *delays* the onset of rapid iron accumulation by about thirty years. Menopause removes this protective mechanism, and due to the presence of lower iron stores, the resulting iron accumulation rate right after menopause may *exceed* the 20-milligram-per-year rate exhibited by men.

Though there is still some quibbling among scientists about the direct link between serum ferritin measurements and iron stores in older people, most now agree that iron accumulation is a fact of life. The results of the Washington State study have been confirmed in other investigations.[7,10] And it is important to keep in mind that the values for excess iron in men and women are only averages: millions of people have far greater iron stores and are at far greater risk for adverse health consequences.

Why Do We Accumulate So Much Iron?

The accumulation of iron as we age may be due to several factors. We tend to lose muscle mass as we age, and perhaps the iron from muscle cells, which remains trapped in the body due to the lack of any excretion mechanism, simply adds to iron stores. Similarly, we may lose the capacity to make enough red blood cells over time, and so some of the iron we needed for hemoglobin goes into storage.[6]

But the dominant factor is excess intake of iron. In most developed countries like the U.S., people eat a lot of meat, which contains easily absorbable iron compared to that in plant foods. And the excess amount that we absorb does not need to be very much to lead to an increased iron burden as we age. For example, the "average man" in the Washington State study absorbed an excess of 20 milligrams of iron per year above that needed to offset his normal losses. If he could prevent this excess absorption, which is equivalent to only .05 milligram of iron per day, he could become iron-balanced, wherein daily iron absorption roughly matches daily losses. You can begin to see how important it is to properly and accurately define your iron intake for life.

Few of Us Are Iron-Balanced

Figure 2-2 puts the iron balance story in a nutshell. For men, absorbed iron normally exceeds iron losses, and true iron balance is rarely achieved. Premenopausal women who are menstruating are the only large group in our country who are likely to be iron-balanced: absorbed iron equals iron losses and the total iron stored away is a comfortable 200–300 milligrams. Postmenopausal women (or younger women who are not menstruating regularly), on the other hand, have an iron status like that of men and are unbalanced iron accumulators.

Birth of the Iron-Accumulator Man

You can see that humans are like iron accumulation machines, roaming the earth in search of more of the metal. If iron were gold, surely we would all be rich! Where did we get this uncanny ability to acquire iron?

Perhaps we can blame the whole problem on plants. (At least *they* cannot talk back!) Over two and a half billion years ago, everything was peachy: the evolution of multicelled organisms was going along fine, aided in part by the marvelous chemical power of abundant iron. The form of iron present then, called ferrous iron, dissolved well in water and was quite accessible. The trouble started when the first green leaf appeared, and photosynthesis, the process by which plants derive their energy from sunlight, began to "pollute" the atmosphere. In the presence of light, plants use water and carbon dioxide, releasing oxygen into the atmosphere. Oxygen, in turn, converts iron to rust, which only sparingly dissolves in water. As vegetation began to cover the globe, other organisms were forced to evolve intricate ways to get enough iron—or die.[11]

The evolutionary pathways that led to the human species brought successive add-on advantages to these primitive strategies for obtaining iron. After all, humans and our primitive cousins needed to store iron away for those long, hungry winters spent in caves. In those days, there was no chance of getting too much iron: you needed as much as you could get. There also was no need to evolve a mechanism to get rid of excess iron because no one lived long enough to accumulate much of it: life spans were only about twenty to forty years.

Today we have virtually the same bodies, but a very different diet. A continuous stream of iron enters our system from readily available meats and iron-enriched foods. Your body responds naturally by hoarding it, waiting for the proverbial rainy day—or hungry winter—that never comes.

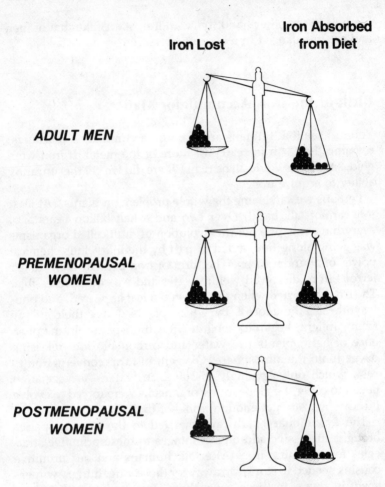

Figure 2-2. Iron balance in adult men and women. This chart summarizes what we know about iron balance in adult men and women. Men absorb more iron from the diet than they lose through sweat, urine, and cells that are shed from the intestinal wall, hair, skin, and nails, resulting in the accumulation of iron as they age. Menstruation keeps younger women iron-balanced; their iron losses are greater than those of men, but this is roughly compensated by the amount of iron they absorb. When the iron losses from menstruation cease at menopause, women become unbalanced iron accumulators.

These iron stores are like water in a camel's hump: we can draw on them at any time in our lives when we are short on iron. In fact, almost all of us could live for long periods of time with no iron in our diet whatsoever. Premenopausal women, who lose an average of 1.6 milligrams of iron per day, could go without iron for roughly three to seven months before depleting their iron stores of 200–300 milligrams. Most men and post-menopausal women could go without iron for two years or more! (This assumes an average daily iron loss of one milligram and iron stores of at least 600 milligrams.)

In these modern times, improved sanitation and health care keep us living longer and longer. As we age, we build up an arsenal of rusty iron that is never called to war. The only attacks it makes are on our own bodies.

Deadly Chemistry

All this rust stored away in your body cannot do you any good. Sure, it's good to have a little storage iron—100–300 milligrams or so, but not the 800 milligrams or more that is present in over half of us. At best, the extra 600 milligrams or so just sits there inside the vast geodesic dome of ferritin: *it has no function in the human body*.

The actual problem begins not with the rusty storage iron itself but with the free iron floating around in our cells. Scientists still do not know a lot about this form of iron. One iron expert, Dr. Robert Crichton of the Université Catholique de Louvain in France, has referred to a "mysterious intermediate pool [of iron] whose nature is about as well characterized as that of the Loch Ness Monster."[12] But it does appear that as the level of stored iron increases, the amount of free iron increases too. This free iron can unleash a destructive chain reaction that makes use of iron's special property of combining with different forms of oxygen. When bound to hemoglobin, iron is a little chemical angel, carefully escorting oxygen in the blood and benevolently delivering it to the neediest tissues. But free—alone and bare—iron is a little devil, a neighborhood brat playing with a dangerous chemistry set and a tank of oxygen. The interaction between iron and oxygen then becomes destructive, and our tissues are the victims.[13,14]

The process is called *oxidation*, and you have seen it now and then when dinner leftovers are not eaten soon enough. Given enough time, fat-containing foods get rancid; so do we.

Iron is known as an excellent catalyst for oxidation. This means it speeds up an otherwise slow chemical reaction. Scientists are still sorting out exactly what happens when free iron and oxygen meet. One possibility is that iron is responsible for the formation of a deadly, highly reactive form of oxygen known as the *hydroxyl radical*. This form of oxygen is like a little touch-sensitive bomb, reacting with almost anything in its path. A second possibility is that the culprit is a molecular dumbbell consisting of one atom of iron and one of oxygen. This compound is thought to be just as dangerous as the hydroxyl radical.

The damage caused by this iron-catalyzed reaction is extensive and not limited to any one particular cell component. Some of the most severe damage occurs to the fatty molecules composing our vital cell walls. A chain reaction in the wall can end up destroying its capacity to communicate with other cells and can cause critical substances to leak out. Other vital targets are hit as well. A growing group of scientists now believe that tissue damage initiated in this fashion is at the core of a wide range of human diseases, including heart disease and cancer, as well as being fundamental to the aging process itself.[14]

Partial Protection

With this type of destructive chemistry always possible, living organisms are really walking time bombs. We have all the necessary ingredients for disaster: fat and iron in our bodies and oxygen from the air. How do we even survive?

We survive as long as we do in part because we possess or consume a number of defensive substances that protect us from oxidizing to death. One class of these substances is known as antioxidants. These include vitamin E, which protects cell walls, and vitamin C, which patrols the interior of the cell. These substances can prevent chain reactions and convert toxic substances into safe ones. Similar compounds, such as butylated hydroxytoluene or BHT, are often added to foods to slow down the oxidation process.

A second important class of protective molecules are specialized enzymes that scavenge toxic forms of oxygen. One of these enzymes, *superoxide dismutase* or SOD, captures an activated form of oxygen known as superoxide. SOD is often billed as the ultimate antioxidant and is actually sold in tablet form at health food stores. However, there is no way that the orally administered SOD could be helpful—the enzyme completely decomposes during digestion. At best, SOD is an expensive protein supplement!

The protection provided by these substances is, unfortunately, insufficient. Megadoses of antioxidants are unlikely to help and, in some cases, may actually exacerbate tissue oxidation. For example, vitamin C increases the availability of iron from storage sites and is known to increase tissue damage in patients with iron overload (see Chapter 17).

Many scientists now believe that stray iron atoms must be sequestered in order to actually prevent oxidation. Your body does attempt to do this by keeping most of the iron firmly bound to proteins. Nevertheless, small amounts of iron still escape and participate in oxidation reactions.

Clearly we have an imperfect iron-control system. Perhaps in human evolution, it was not necessary to develop a better system. Since high iron levels are only reached in middle and old age, the physiological consequences did not affect reproductive capacity and thus would not be a factor in evolution.

Iron and You

Probably the best way to control iron is simply to minimize the total amount stored in your body. This is the heart of the Iron Balance Health Plan. No drugs, no megadoses of vitamins—just common sense. The evidence supporting the plan is presented in Parts 3 and 4.

But first let us take a closer look at the social and medical factors that led to the high iron levels in our bodies today. Now that you know the facts about human iron metabolism—most important, how we accumulate iron as we age—you have to wonder why iron *deficiency* is such a highly publicized problem in America and why iron *excess* is rarely mentioned. The answers to these questions are in Part 2.

Part 2

ARE YOU *REALLY* ANEMIC?

The Myth of "Iron-Poor Blood" in America

3

The Geritol Scam

Madge feels tired all the time. The TV commercials and women's magazines tell her that she might be anemic. She goes to see her doctor. Her doctor tests her blood-iron level and finds she's a little low. Madge goes home with some iron supplements.

What's wrong with this scenario? Madge isn't really anemic. In fact she may have the healthiest iron level in the world! In addition, the iron supplement may, over time, do her harm. And her *actual* problem—perhaps a viral or yeast infection, stress, or depression—may never be discovered.

What is going on?

A not so funny thing has happened on our way to the twenty-first century in preventative health care and nutrition. You would have thought by now—when open-heart surgery and hip replacements are commonplace, when our understanding of molecular biology is rapidly accelerating, when miracle drugs can extend life—that scientists could agree on the optimal amount of iron that should be present in the human body. You might also have expected that iron-deficiency anemia, one of mankind's oldest and simplest maladies, would be so well characterized by now that physicians would at least agree on how to diagnose it, and on how low iron levels should be before treatment is required.

As it turns out, the steady progress in our knowledge of crucial nutrients has, in the case of iron, been derailed by clever drug and food advertising, and by overzealous nutritionists, politicians, and public health authorities. These forces have constantly exaggerated the prevalence of iron-deficiency anemia and underplayed the dangers of iron excess. As shown by the example of Madge at the beginning of this chapter, the result of this distortion is that people have unnecessarily consumed far too much iron in the form of prescriptions, over-the-counter supplements, and iron-fortified foods.

How did this all get started? A good place to begin is at the J. B. Williams Company, the original makers of the popular multivitamin and iron supplement Geritol.

A Snake Oil for "Tired Blood"

J. B. Williams, based in New York City, was one of the smaller drug companies, the kind that executives at larger firms buy and sell over lunch. Their products were decidedly low-tech: they made Aqua Velva and Lectric Shave, as well as over-the-counter remedies like Sominex and Geritol. Market share for these products is obtained only through relentless advertising, and Williams was very good at this. Unlike other drug firms, they even owned their own ad agency. It was reported that in 1962 alone they spent $3.5 million on Geritol advertising (equal to about $20 million today, adjusted for inflation).[1]

In the 1950s, the talented ad executives at Williams were trying to figure out how to sell millions of bottles of Geritol to the American public. Geritol is a simple nutritional supplement, a solution or tablet containing small quantities of a few vitamins and a lot of iron, the featured ingredient.

The ad executives eventually hit upon an idea that was to add new terms to the American lexicon and distort the proper role of iron in our diet. Instead of selling Geritol for what it was—a nutritional supplement—they would sell it as a quick-fix remedy for fatigue, a known symptom of true iron deficiency. Though the medical establishment knew that in all likelihood fatigue is caused by many conditions other than iron deficiency, the public did not. What notions of iron the public did have—the connotations of strength and the connection to Popeye's spinach— would make Geritol synonymous with strength and vitality.

One group targeted by J. B. Williams was older Americans— those more likely to feel tired. By using the prefix *Geri-*, for *geriatric*, the company was pushing iron to one of the groups that need it least. As you read in Chapter 2, most adult men and postmenopausal women accumulate iron and have more than sufficient iron stores.

As you may recall, the company's ads also focused a great deal on women, purporting that Geritol would improve their lives. Following is the script of a television ad from the early 1960s, in which Art Linkletter holds a bottle of Geritol and says:[1]

> The other day I heard a lady say, "I feel so tired every night, a team of horses couldn't drag me out!" If you feel too tired even to go out and have a little fun, that worn-out feeling may be due to iron-poor blood. And if you've been taking vitamins, yet *still* feel tired, remember, *vitamins alone* can't build up iron-poor blood. But GERITOL can! Because just two GERITOL tablets or two tablespoons of GERITOL liquid contain seven vitamins *plus twice* the iron in a pound of calves' liver.
>
> In only one day GERITOL-iron is in your bloodstream carrying *strength* and *energy* to every part of your body. Check with your doctor, and if you've been feeling worn out because of iron-poor blood and especially after a cold, the flu, or sore throat, take GERITOL *every day*.
>
> *Feel stronger fast* in just seven days or your money back from the GERITOL folks. [Italics included in actual script.]

In another ad from that period, a mother takes a break from straightening her boy's room and reflects, "I feel so tired and run-down lately. I wonder what the trouble is?" The booming announcer then exclaims, "*Your* trouble may be due to iron-deficiency anemia. We call it *TIRED BLOOD*."[1]

Geritol v. the Federal Trade Commission

Not many people knew then—and even fewer know today—that the Geritol ad campaign was illegal. The Federal Trade Commission, which is supposed to protect consumers from fraudulent ads, began in 1959 a well-meant but largely ineffective seventeen-year battle with J. B. Williams.[1-6] In 1963, the commission held extensive hearings at which thirty-nine prominent physicians and experts in iron metabolism lambasted the Geritol claims. It was agreed that, in the great majority of people, fatigue was not caused by iron deficiency, and therefore Geritol was not an appropriate remedy. One paid witness for the company even admitted that if a person begins to feel better within a few hours after taking the product, "Obviously, this is the placebo effect."[1] (A placebo is a pill containing no active medicine; the "placebo effect" occurs when a patient is fooled into thinking this inactive medicine actually alleviated the problem.)

In 1965, the Federal Trade Commission finally issued a cease-and-desist order to prevent the company from airing the commercials. Unfortunately, a lot of damage had already been done: Americans had heard the misleading commercials for more than six years while the commission was slowly collecting the evidence. "Iron-poor blood" was etched in almost everyone's mind.

The response of the J. B. Williams Company was truly remarkable—and gutsy. Though the executives buried a few clarifying words in the new scripts, they extended their claims to even broader but more subtle themes. Now Geritol would not only make you feel better, but it would also improve your sex life and marriage. In one of the new ads, entitled "Man Coming Home," the potion is almost sold as a sex tonic. In the opinion of some, the commercials also began to cross the boundaries of good taste. This is the way the Federal Trade Commission later described the company's belligerence, using this one ad as an example:[1]

The commercials broadcast for Geritol since the [cease-and-desist] order . . . are no less objectionable than the [original] commercials. . . . Five of the eight commercials . . . depict the transformation of a wan, lackadaisical housewife into a veritable tigress.

Typical of these five is the commercial entitled "Man Coming Home." This depicts a smiling husband entering his home, where he is dismayed by the sight of his wife. She is in curlers, tired-looking and leaning against the doorway. Moreover, the kitchen appears to have been untouched for some time, being strewn with unwashed pots and pans. The husband, feigning anger, draws a pistol from his jacket and fires it at his now apprehensive wife. From the pistol emerges a flag reading "Iron-poor tired blood? Try Geritol." A card reading "later" appears on the television screen, followed by the same setting but with remarkable differences. The household is spotless. The haggard-looking woman seen at the beginning of the commercial now is attractively coiffured and made up, and in the wording of the script for this commercial, "garbed in a slinky gown." Her husband enters to find her so attired and posing against the piano with "a 'come hither' expression" and a rose in her mouth. She literally sweeps her husband off his feet by embracing him passionately and enthusiastically, as the commercial ends with the words "Feel stronger fast" appearing on the screen, and the audio portion of the commercial advising the viewer that "If you're tired because of iron-poor blood, Geritol can help *you* feel stronger fast. Maybe not *this* fast. But fast."

Subsequent Geritol ads continued on the theme of improved marital union, with the now famous line, "My wife, I think I'll keep her." It is worth mentioning that the ad executives at J. B. Williams were doing something similar with another of their low-tech products as well: ads for Vivarin, a cheap stimulant that was simply dextrose and an amount of caffeine equivalent to two cups of coffee, were also attacked by the Federal Trade Commission as false and misleading, particularly in regard to indirect sexual- or marital-improvement claims.[1] One ad started off with a housewife's remarkable discovery: "One day it dawned on me that I was boring my husband to death. . . ."

Round Two

At the time this was happening, the consumer activist movement in the U.S. was beginning to build strength. In the summer of 1968, Ralph Nader sent a team of investigative law students to check up on the Federal Trade Commission. "Nader's Raiders," whom a big-business supporter described as "seven Ivy League students in search of a meaningful summer,"[2] understandably encountered a great deal of resistance but nevertheless managed to collect enough information to produce an important document: *The Nader Report on the Federal Trade Commission*. This report included a discussion of the Commission's mishandling of the Geritol case:[3]

> For thirty years Geritol has been permitted to lie blatantly to Americans, telling us that we should buy and take Geritol if we feel run-down or listless. The fact is that the number of people with these symptoms who would be helped by Geritol is almost infinitesimal. Yet these symptoms are indicative of a number of other afflictions, afflictions that should lead one immediately to a physician, not to a bottle of substantially useless Geritol. . . .
>
> In 1967, after years of "investigation" and litigation, the FTC ordered the J. B. Williams Company, the manufacturer of Geritol, to stop misrepresenting the product as a generally effective remedy for fatigue. In spite of this order, later affirmed by the Court of Appeals, Geritol's TV advertisements have changed little in emphasis, as most viewers well know. . . .
>
> Having discovered a clear violation of an outstanding cease-and-desist order, did the Commission announce that it would seek "civil penalties" against Geritol's makers? No, it merely warned them to stop "flouting" the order and to

file by January 31, 1969, a report showing what steps were being taken to tone down the commercials. . . .

The new commercials still contained substantial misrepresentations. Yet, the Commission did nothing. Meanwhile, Geritol . . . has gone back to the more extreme and blatant deceptions—tying tiredness, the medical profession, and health to a product that has very little connection with any of them. One may well ask what lesson other companies condemned under FTC orders will learn from the highly visible Geritol case.

In his preface to the report, Ralph Nader described the motivations of the company and its powerful Washington law firm—which was running up a lot of "billable hours"—stating that they "have little to lose by these delays (even after being cited for violations of the order) and much to gain—continuing sales to people misled into believing that Geritol can make them healthier."

Finally, in 1970, the Justice Department filed a $1 million suit against J. B. Williams, charging that the company violated Federal Trade Commission orders to stop deceptive advertising for Geritol and FemIron, a related product for women. The story made headlines, with *The New York Times* headline proclaiming GERITOL SUED OVER 'TIRED BLOOD.'[4] The big-business supporter, *The Wall Street Journal*, started its article by belittling the government: "Perhaps a little tired and irritable, the Federal Government went into the courts in its eleven-year-long dispute over advertising claims for Geritol."[5] J. B. Williams responded smugly with the standard press release: "We have every confidence that the courts will find no basis for this charge."[5]

They were wrong. In 1973 another *Wall Street Journal* article on the Geritol saga began, "Some people at J. B. Williams Co. might have 'that run-down feeling' this morning."[5] A district court judge had found that the company's "conduct amounted to gross negligence and bordered on recklessness," and she levied fines totaling $812,000, at that time the largest ever for Federal Trade Commission violations.

The company's lawyers worked hard to stretch out the conflict and diminish its impact on the product and the company's image. They got an appeals court to send the case back to a district court for what would be a lengthy jury trial. Finally, in 1976, they had managed to chisel the $812,000 fine down to a total of $302,000 for advertising violations with both Geritol and FemIron, and the case was settled out of court. Though this was still, at the time, the largest award for deceptive advertising, the company did not have to admit that it was guilty of violating the original Federal Trade Commission order.[4,5]

Geritol Today

Certainly a Nader's Raider today would have to conclude in hindsight that the struggle against Geritol was largely lost. The commercials became part of American culture, and Geritol became a very successful product. As the J. B. Williams Company was purchased by Nabisco in 1972 and then by the British company Beecham Group Ltd. in 1982, Geritol has always been an important part of the Williams arsenal. It, along with a new version called Geritol Complete, is now sold by the Consumer Brands division of the newly merged drug company SmithKline Beecham.

The package inserts for Geritol and Geritol Complete continue to promulgate half truths and potentially dangerous recommendations:

> With your purchase of this bottle of Geritol you have taken an important step forward in the treatment and prevention of iron poor blood—America's #1 nutritional problem.

Wrong. As you will learn in the next chapter, the prevalence of iron deficiency has been grossly exaggerated in this country. Iron deficiency is not the "number-one nutritional problem"; our biggest problem is *overconsumption* of fat, cholesterol, and other substances, rather than *underconsumption* of iron.

> Take just one tablespoonful of Geritol daily and its uniquely rich iron formula will give you 5 times the minimum daily requirement of iron. No other leading supple-

ment gives you that much iron in one dose. That's why we
say *iron* is Geritol's middle name.

Take iron-rich Geritol every day. . . .

Since you saw in Chapter 2 that most of us accumulate a storehouse of iron as we age, the massive amounts of iron in Geritol
are far too much to be taking in every day. This will only hasten
the accumulation process, possibly leading to adverse health
effects.

Can men take Geritol Complete? Yes. Geritol Complete
provides sound nutritional protection for both men and
women, although men do not usually need as much iron
as women.

It is nice of the company to acknowledge the well-known fact
that men do not have as hard a time getting enough iron as
women. But what is not mentioned is that almost all adult men
have already accumulated more iron than they can ever use,
and they gain nothing—except the added health risk—by adding to this storehouse of iron.

One Small Step (Backward) for Mankind

The Geritol scam sensitized the nation to iron deficiency. No
matter how objective and knowledgeable you were, those in-
cessant commercials had their effect. Our cultural notions of iron
and its connotations of strength prepared us to be duped by the
J. B. Williams Company. (One wonders why they did not use
Popeye in some of their ads.) As a result, millions of people
needlessly consumed unnecessary iron supplements.

A sensible approach to iron nutrition, based on the facts about
iron accumulation and the potential dangers thereof, became
even more unlikely in this country when the federal government
began to promulgate the myth of epidemic iron deficiency. While

some of us can consciously try to ignore television commercials, it is considerably more difficult to disbelieve our leaders. In the next chapter you will see how politicians and nutrition experts distorted the truth about iron and set this country back more than twenty years in reaching a sound policy regarding this important but potentially dangerous nutrient.

4

Politics and the Mismeasuring of Anemia

In the late 1960s, two well-meaning senators "discovered" a serious problem in America: malnutrition of the poor. In their zeal to bring this problem to the public's attention and raise tax dollars to alleviate it, they started a snowball that eventually rolled right over our national nutritional policy regarding iron.

Against the backdrop of heavy Geritol advertising, more people than ever would be led to believe that they had "iron-poor blood," and that iron supplements were the cure. We may never know the overall impact on the health of Americans, including the harm done to a million or so people who were already overloaded with iron.

This is the heart of America's iron story, a story of rough-and-ready politicians, nutritionists eager to be in the public eye, and national nutrition surveys that appeared to be based more on politics than on science.

Hunger "Discovered"

In March 1967 Senators Joseph Clark and Robert Kennedy of the Senate Labor Committee's Subcommittee on Poverty heard testimony concerning the plight of poverty-stricken blacks in the Mississippi Delta.[1-3] The subject of food availability dominated the hearing after one expert testified that people were "going around begging just to feed their children." Even a conservative Republican senator reacted to this news, promising to bring this "emergency" to President Johnson's attention. Clark and Kennedy saw an opportunity both to upstage their conservative colleague and to focus the nation's attention on a problem only the Democratic party could solve.

Kennedy said, "I want to see it," and he and Clark arranged a personal tour of dilapidated shacks and the forgotten poor in the Delta. After seeing the appalling conditions, Kennedy tried to control his emotions in plain sight of the press and said, "I'm going back to Washington to do something about this." Since, as one reporter put it, "Robert Kennedy was news," hunger in America had made the front page.

This one event and its extensive press coverage gave enormous impetus to the "hunger lobby." A number of reports and exposés, including the powerful 1969 CBS documentary *Hunger in America*, told the shocking truth: a modern nation with routine food surpluses was not feeding its own citizens.

Soon the hunger lobby needed new leadership. In early 1968, Kennedy was busy campaigning for the presidency, a campaign that would end tragically with his assassination. The gauntlet fell to another liberal Democrat, Senator George McGovern from South Dakota. Though not as charismatic as Kennedy, McGovern was nonetheless successful in rallying attention to the malnutrition issue. He successfully fought for the establishment of an important new congressional committee, the Senate Select Committee on Nutrition and Human Needs.

With the election of Richard Nixon as president in 1968, McGovern and other liberals on his new committee had their work cut out for them. Skeptics had thought that the initial reports of malnutrition were anecdotal and exaggerated, and a Republican administration would be unlikely to offer much help to overcome them. As a McGovern biographer, Robert Anson, put it, the committee got its "first break" on January 20, 1969, two days after Nixon took office, with the release of some "hard" numbers: the preliminary results of a large national survey.[3]

The Ten State Nutrition Survey

It was the Ten State Nutrition Survey that gave the impetus to nutritionists, doctors, and drug companies to overestimate the prevalence of "iron-poor blood" in America. Iron-deficiency anemia was one of the chief targets of the study. Unfortunately, the "hard" numbers on anemia were highly misinterpreted and exaggerated for years to come. The survey did much for the well-meaning hunger lobby, but at the same time it promulgated erroneous notions about iron that have not been fully corrected to this day.

It was supposed to be the best nutrition survey ever conducted. When it was finally completed, over 86,000 people had been interviewed. About half of them underwent a basic clinical examination, including a blood test. The ten states studied included those with average family incomes both higher—California, Massachusetts, Michigan, New York, and Washington—and lower—Kentucky, Louisiana, South Carolina, Texas, and West Virginia—than the national average.[4]

Playing the Numbers Game

It is particularly revealing to take a critical look at the results of the Ten State survey pertaining to the prevalence of anemia. In the analysis of the data, men were classified as having "low" hemoglobin readings if they had fewer than 14 grams of hemoglobin per 100 milliliters of blood (one milliliter is equal to one cubic centimeter); for women the cutoff was set at 12 grams per 100 milliliters. The percentage of adults with "low" readings, presumably as a result of iron deficiency, is shown in the table below for both white and black subjects:

Percentage of Subjects with "Low" Hemoglobin Levels in Low-Income States (Ten State Nutrition Survey, 1968–1970)

	MALES (cutoff 14 g/100 ml)		FEMALES (cutoff 12 g/100 ml)	
Age Group	White	Black	White	Black
17–44	20.7%	43.7%	16.0%	39.4%
45–49	22.0%	53.0%	10.2%	26.8%

These results are remarkable—and suspect—for two reasons. First, these are *very* high prevalence numbers; could this many people really be low on iron? Secondly, in all four age-race categories, men were observed to have a greater prevalence of mild anemia than women. This is ludicrous; women are more likely to have mild anemia due to iron loss in the monthly menstrual cycle. Dr. William Crosby, now the director of hematology at the Chapman Cancer Center in Joplin, Missouri, and one of the clearest thinkers in the anemia field, responded to the results in an editorial published in the *Journal of the American Medical Association*:[5]

> [The survey found] that 22 percent of the men tested had iron-deficiency anemia. The report did not point out that men do not get iron-deficiency anemia unless they have blood loss. Are 22 percent of American men bleeding?
>
> To nutritionists these figures have indicated something dreadfully wrong with the national diet. To physicians they indicate something dreadfully wrong with the Ten-State Survey.

What was wrong, of course, was the arbitrary cutoff values. First, they were set too high. It was unlikely that 10–53 percent of the population in one of the richest countries of the world was anemic. If one applied lower cutoff values to the data, considerably lower prevalence estimates resulted.

Second, though the cutoff values chosen were nice even numbers, the relative values for men and women were inappropriately set, resulting in the higher prevalence estimates for men. These results from the Ten State survey reveal how arbitrary cutoffs can lead to misinterpretations. As we will see in the next chapter, many experts have questioned the use of these cutoffs in trying to assess the prevalence of iron deficiency.

When the preliminary findings of the study were reported to McGovern's Senate committee in January 1969, none of these subtleties were discussed. To dramatize the findings, the numbers for children were emphasized. One of the most widely quoted results was that 34 percent of the poor children were "badly anemic."[3] Though it is well known that children can be more susceptible to iron deficiency, this particular result is distorted. Often it was not mentioned that this value was for black children in low-income states. More important, as shown in the preceding table and discussed in several treatises on anemia, blacks at any given income level may naturally have lower hemoglobin levels than whites because of inherited differences in their metabolism. This of course does not make them anemic by any means.[6]

Nonetheless, the word that anemia was rampant in America had already gotten out. The extensive press coverage of Kennedy's hunger "discovery" and the Ten State survey focused on initial results rather than a careful, scientific analysis. In a way, the situation paralleled the Geritol scam, where misleading commercials were shown for years before finally being pulled off the air. Of course, in the case of the Ten State survey, it was our government, not some drug company, that had put its stamp of approval on the anemia myth.

The NHANES Survey: An Improved Version of the Ten State?

The second set of large surveys in the U.S. would be designed from the conservative perspective of the Nixon administration.[7] Perhaps it was the Republican approach, or perhaps the ap-

proach of any administration that did not want embarrassing
questions raised.

The Nixon administration had tried to squelch the effect of
the revelations about hunger, and many of its members were
frankly skeptical about the findings. In deciding how to respond
to the Ten State results and the hunger lobby's success, White
House notes reveal that the president himself told the Secretary
of Health, Education, and Welfare:[3]

> You can say that this administration will have the first
> complete, far-ranging attack on the problem of hunger in
> history. Use all the rhetoric, so long as it doesn't cost any
> money.

The responsibility for the new survey was split between the
Department of Health, Education, and Welfare's National Center
for Health Statistics, which would direct the work, and the Center for Disease Control in Atlanta, which would perform the
laboratory analysis. With the power split between two distant
groups, *no* results would be available until three to five years
after the onset of data collection: a comfortable timetable for
those who faced periodic reelection trauma.

The Nixon administration also changed the name of the survey
to the National Health and Nutrition Examination Survey
(NHANES). At an estimated cost of at least $4 million a year,
NHANES I was conducted between 1971 and 1974 and NHANES
II between 1976 and 1980. NHANES II is thought to be the most
comprehensive health survey ever conducted. Over 20,000 people, aged six months to 74 years, were examined and interviewed
in sixty-four locations throughout the U.S.[7]

Over the last ten years, the data from NHANES II have provided the raw material for numerous important epidemiological
studies relating to nutrition and disease incidence. But, despite
the use of hemoglobin measurements and no less than three
indices of iron status, its analysis in this area was still based on
arbitrary cutoff values, and it left many questions unanswered.

In the analysis of NHANES II data, a person having two or
three "abnormal" iron readings was classified as having "im-

paired iron status." The table below shows the percentage of adults found to have this "disease":[8,9]

Percentage of Subjects With "Impaired Iron Status" (NHANES II, 1976–1980)

Age	Males	Females
15–19	0.1%	14.2%
20–44	0.6%	9.6%
45–64	1.9%	4.8%

One gratifying result from this analysis of the NHANES II data is that, compared to the dubious interpretations of the Ten State study, the iron status of men now appeared okay, with less than 2 percent of men lacking in iron.

Women, on the other hand, showed appreciable iron-deficiency rates of 5–15 percent, not unlike those found in the Ten State study. However, a closer look at the data once again reveals some annoying discrepancies. For a large number of the women, independent measurements of blood hemoglobin levels did not seem linked to the result of the iron test. For example, 31 percent of those women considered anemic (those with hemoglobin readings less than 11.9 grams per 100 milliliters of blood) had perfectly normal iron levels, whereas 22 percent of the nonanemic women had at least one "abnormal" iron reading.[8,9] This overlap between the "healthy" and "iron impaired" subjects again brings up the question of how to define an iron-related disease state. Are ten million women really sick?

Falling Short of the RDA

The myth that iron deficiency is extremely prevalent among women has been compounded by food consumption surveys which repeatedly show low iron intakes for women. Since 1943, the recommended dietary allowance of various nutrients for the different age and sex subgroups in our population has been determined by a private group of scientists, the Food and Nutrition Board of the National Academy of Sciences. Usually, the highest value required for any of the subgroups is then designated as the U.S. Recommended Daily Allowance (RDA) by the Department of Agriculture. It is these overall RDAs that are used in calculating the nutritional information on food labels.

You should realize that the RDAs are *not* minimums, and therefore people ingesting somewhat lower quantities of any nutrient are unlikely to develop deficiency diseases. Also a lot of guesswork goes on in the determination of the RDAs: humans are complex and variable organisms, and quantitative nutrition has got to be one of our most complex sciences. Scientists have vastly different opinions about the appropriate levels of many nutrients. The publication of the latest version of the RDAs was held up for many years because of such disagreement.

The 1980 RDA for iron is 10 milligrams for men and 18 for women. The logic behind these numbers is very simple. Since men lose about one milligram of iron per day and absorb only about 10 percent of the iron in the foods they eat, they will need to consume 10 milligrams of iron each day to make up for the one milligram lost. It is assumed that premenopausal women lose an additional .8 milligram a day, on average, due to the monthly menstrual cycle. Thus, using the same 10 percent absorption factor, the RDA for women was set at 18 milligrams.

Do we actually get these amounts in our diet? The National Food Consumption Survey (NFCS), conducted in 1977 and 1978 by the U.S. Department of Agriculture, is the largest and most recent source of information on this subject. The NFCS examined three-day nutrient intake in approximately 36,000 people in the U.S. Men were found to have adequate iron intake, but more than 80 percent of women failed to fulfill their RDA for iron.[10] It is numbers like these that have kept the myth of "iron-poor blood" going strong.

What is wrong with these consumption surveys and their conclusions? Plenty. First, in the special case of iron, they do not take into account that any iron absorbed in excess of a person's *actual* requirements on a given day is stored away for later use. As discussed in Chapter 2, this storage iron usually increases throughout a person's life, decreasing the real requirement for iron. Secondly, there are vast differences in nutritional requirements among individuals, due to inherent factors in our bodies or differences in behavior. Women who use oral contraceptives, for example, have lower menstrual blood losses and, consequently, lower iron requirements. Third, there are a lot of problems with the surveys themselves related to how the data are obtained, including factors such as the skill of the interviewer and the memory of the subject.

It is amusing that in the most recent edition of the RDA tables (the tenth edition, published in 1989; see Appendix A), the Food and Nutrition Board decreased the iron RDA for women from 18 to 15 milligrams. (In 1992, the Food and Drug Administration will replace the U.S. RDA for labeling purposes with Reference Daily Intake [RDI] values; the RDI for iron will then be set at 15 milligrams.) The reasoning of the experts was that the percentage of iron absorbed from meals, normally about 10 percent, increases in women with depleted iron stores; the original RDA did not take this into account. In addition, they felt that the 18 milligrams per day was very difficult to obtain and 15 milligrams should be more than sufficient.[11] This is at least a step in the right direction: the RDA of 18 milligrams was clearly too high since the 80 percent of women who fail to get their RDA of iron were not showing up at their doctors' offices with true anemia.

Shadows Behind the Myth

Between the highly charged hunger issue and the misinterpreted surveys, our government was never able to establish a sound nutritional policy regarding iron. In this, the American people have been poorly served. While attempting to solve the nutritional problems of a few, activists never adequately considered the effect of their efforts on the bulk of Americans, whose diets were adequate, if not excessive.

The effect of this overemphasis on deficiencies might be negligible for most nutrients. But in the case of iron, a classic double-edged nutrient that accumulates within us, great damage can be done. As you will see in Chapter 6, many nutritionists have constantly overlooked the potential dangers of raising the entire population's iron levels through massive food fortification campaigns. One critic referred to these efforts as "an uncontrolled experiment on the entire American population." In the case of iron, we may never know precisely the extent of health effects from overconsumption. In addition, the emphasis on iron deficiency made it very difficult to alert doctors as to the prevalence of iron overload. As a result, thousands of iron-overload victims have gone undetected for years while iron was destroying their bodies.

In the next chapter, we take a look at how the myth of "iron-poor blood" in America still influences patient care in our highly advanced health care system.

5

Anemia Today: Overdiagnosed and Overtreated

Let us return to Madge's trip to the doctor's office and analyze what happens in light of what we now know about this country's distorted view of iron and anemia. You were first introduced to Madge at the beginning of Chapter 3. She was feeling a little "run down" and wanted to know if she was anemic like the television commercials and women's magazines were telling her.

According to Dr. Richard Podell, author of *Doctor, Why Am I So Tired?*, over ten million people visit their doctors every year to find the cause of their fatigue.[1] In many cases, this is probably one of the most difficult questions a doctor can address. Apart from those doctors that dismiss the importance of fatigue and related symptoms—"It's all in your head"—the well-meaning physicians face the daunting challenge of surveying an overwhelming number of potential causes, from serious physical factors such as glandular deficiencies or circulatory disorders to mental conditions—stress or depression—abuse of caffeine, nicotine, or alcohol, or viral or yeast infections. Patients should be prepared for several visits to perhaps more than one doctor to really nail down the cause. Even then, they may achieve nothing

53

more than a little peace of mind coming from the knowledge that the problem is not serious.

Iron deficiency should be at the bottom of the list of potential causes of fatigue. For example, in his 250-page book on fatigue, Dr. Podell devotes only a couple of pages to the importance of iron and other minerals. Unfortunately, as you will see, iron deficiency is "popular" and easy to treat; consequently, it is a favored diagnosis of many doctors.

Madge has done one thing right. Going to see the doctor was an excellent step. For every person who takes this prudent step there are probably five to ten others who resort to dangerous self-medication. Our culture reveres quick-fix remedies such as Geritol or megavitamins, many of which are no better for us than snake oil and, over time, could do us harm. Madge has rightfully rejected these remedies and is not willing to take her health into her own hands.

Instead she puts her health into the hands of her family physician. The doctor listens intently to her complaints and, finding nothing obviously wrong, orders simple blood tests. These include a hemoglobin and possibly a serum iron measurement, but not a somewhat more expensive serum ferritin check. Thus, at best, the doctor will know how much iron is in the blood at the time of the test—this amount varies throughout the day—but will *not* have any idea about the milligrams upon milligrams of iron stored away in Madge's liver, spleen, and bone marrow.

A few tablespoons of blood and a couple days later, Madge gets her diagnosis: mild iron-deficiency anemia. It turns out that she has a hemoglobin reading that is slightly lower than the accepted cutoff value. And, in addition, her serum iron reading is at the low end of the normal range.

The doctor, who is confronted with far more complex and life-threatening cases, is quite pleased with such a simple diagnosis—and with such a simple treatment: iron supplements. He has seen it work so many times in the past: the patient starts taking the pills, the hemoglobin reading jumps up into the normal range and the patient feels great. He thinks to himself, "Maybe this is not such a bad profession after all."

Madge is happy too. She breathes a sigh of relief as she

watches the doctor write out the time-honored prescription for ferrous sulphate: no more tests, no more needles, just some pretty pink pills. She is looking forward to feeling better.

Madge is well prepared to be "cured" by one of the most effective medicines used for ages: the placebo. At least in her case, according to conventional wisdom (however flawed), the doctor had a reason for giving her the supplements: her slightly low hemoglobin reading justified this measure. But iron is prescribed improperly far too often. In a recent survey of 265 family physicians in England, nearly three-quarters of the respondents admitted that they often treated patients with extremely mild anemia with iron supplements, despite the fact that the patients lacked any clinical symptoms of anemia and had hemoglobin readings within the normal range. Up to 40 percent of the doctors also admitted prescribing iron for nonspecific complaints (fatigue, for example) or because the patients requested it.[2]

In the view of some doctors, iron-deficiency anemia is one of the five most *over*diagnosed diseases today.[3] And no wonder: it is so easy to treat. Just add iron and sit back. You can easily see the joy that doctors get from this charade by reading textbooks and articles in medical reviews. One expert writes, "Treatment of iron deficiency is one of the most satisfying experiences in medical practice."

As the placebo effect kicks in, patients will convince themselves they feel better for some period of time. But many of them will be back at the doctor's office with their original complaints soon after. Worse, some of them will take the cue from their doctor's tendency and medicate themselves with even more iron or other drugs. In this case, the original cause of their complaint may never be discovered.

Where Does Anemia Begin and Good Health End?

The real problem begins with the definition of iron-deficiency anemia. Conventionally trained doctors see the lower cutoff for normal hemoglobin readings as 11.9 or 12 grams per 100 milliliters for women and 13 for men. Similarly, arbitrary cutoff values are also used for other tests for anemia. People who have readings below such cutoff values are often judged sick despite the absence of clear symptoms or work impairment. Iron-deficiency anemia is, today, often an imaginary disease!

A handful of doctors have voiced their objections to this simple and somewhat aggressive approach. One of these physicians, Dr. Peter Elwood, an iron-deficiency expert and director of Britain's Medical Research Council Epidemiology Unit in Cardiff, has written:[4]

> The exact definition of iron deficiency has been argued in detail. It would seem, however, that the only reasonable and useful definition of a condition such as this would be based on valid evidence of harm to health or function which can be removed by treatment. One should not base the definition of a condition on some arbitrary level of a biochemical or haematological variate, the relevance of which to health has not been fully worked out. Diagnoses which are based on theoretical concepts of what is ideal are unlikely to be useful and may be misleading.

There is no disagreement about the definition of severe anemia and its clinical symptoms: extremely low hemoglobin and iron levels will impair oxygen delivery to your tissues. In this condition, it wouldn't take more than a flight of stairs to get you really huffing. Even though you probably live at an elevation of zero to 2000 feet, you would feel as if you had just been dropped off at the top of some 12,000-foot mountain where the air is extremely thin. You might get throbbing headaches, also a sign of altitude sickness.

The disagreement is in the "gray area" of mild iron deficiency and slightly reduced hemoglobin readings, like that observed for Madge.[4] In this intermediate zone, the main effect scientists have demonstrated is a reduction in *maximal* work performance.[5] That is, though you could perform all your normal tasks or exercise with no problem, you may not be able to go the extra yard and set a personal record for the time it takes to shovel the snow off the sidewalk or run five miles. I believe that, for most of us, this has little importance. Unless you are an athlete or a manual laborer with an extremely heavy workload, you would never notice any effect on your "performance."

Scientists have also searched for other physical effects of mild iron deficiency. Many of these investigators have postulated that the amount of certain iron-containing enzymes may decrease as the iron supply decreases. The reduction in the concentration of these substances could even occur, they guess, before hemoglobin levels are decreased. This might independently contribute to decreased work capacity, since some of these substances are important in burning fuel at maximum capacity. Other possible effects, such as a decrease in the ability of our immune system to attack invading organisms, are still being debated.[5,6]

Now please keep in mind that iron deficiency should *always* be prevented in certain vulnerable groups in our population, especially infants and children. Iron is crucial for growth and the development of mental capacities. Pregnant women also need plenty of iron, both for the growing fetus and for the newly expanded blood supply. These issues, including what to do if your doctor says you are anemic, are discussed further in Chapter 15.

But for the rest of us, a mild "anemic" state with satisfactory iron stores of 100–300 milligrams is harmless and may protect us against several diseases (see Part 4). Even if there are slight effects on physical work performance, the low-iron state may be healthiest.

Anemia As a Symptom, Not a Disease

A final word on the doctor's response to mild anemia in patients is germane. Blood experts believe that a true anemic state should be more valuable to the doctor as a symptom rather than a disease.[4,7] Markedly abnormal hemoglobin readings should tell the doctor that the patient is most likely losing considerable amounts of blood at some remote site in the body. Ulcers, colon cancer, and other potentially life-threatening diseases are often the source of the bleeding. (In most of these cases, the blood gets metabolized in the gastrointestinal tract and is often hidden in the stool.) The earlier these conditions are caught, the better. Simply prescribing iron pills will get rid of the anemia, but it essentially covers up this important diagnostic indicator for serious disease. In fact, several hematologists have objected to excess fortification of foods with iron, since this would raise the iron levels in the population, "masking" the appearance of anemia in those individuals with serious conditions.

In this chapter you have seen how the anemia myth has penetrated the doctor's office and led to the overtreatment of iron deficiency. Now let us turn from the doctor's office to the grocery store and look at nonprescription sources of iron in our high-iron society.

6

Fortification Follies

Enriched. Isn't that a nice word to see on food labels? It seems like you're getting even more than you paid for: you're becoming "enriched" in nutrients!

There is no problem as far as I know with adding vitamins to our flour, bread, cereal, and milk. The problem is with excessive iron fortification. As you know from Chapter 2, most of us are already "rich" in iron and can get by on far less than our RDA. We don't need more iron than is already present naturally in our food.

Nonetheless, many of the forces behind the anemia-in-America myth have long believed we need to add more iron to the American diet to decrease the prevalence of this "epidemic." These evangelists had their most visible clash with the proponents of common sense and caution over a proposal to increase the amount of iron in common foodstuffs like wheat flour and bread. This confrontation marks an important stage in the evolution of public health policies toward iron. The questions it raised were important to the health of millions of individuals: Should the government legislate an increase in iron content that might raise the iron levels of most Americans? Would the health risks outweigh the benefits of helping a few iron-deficient people?

Iron for the People

Following the first Nationwide Food Consumption Survey in 1936–1937, President Franklin Roosevelt called for a National Nutrition Conference in 1941 to focus attention on deficiencies in the nation's food supply. The first RDAs were issued, and with the support of the American Medical Association, the National Academy of Sciences, and the food industry, the Food and Drug Administration (FDA) set new standards for enriched flour and bread.[1,2] Iron and the B-complex vitamins thiamine, riboflavin, and niacin were added back to processed grain products to prerefinement, or "natural," levels. With the growing awareness of the importance of micronutrients, no one had any objections to this action. (It could be argued, however, that the chemical form of the enrichment iron was not identical to that in whole wheat.)

During the 1960s, the FDA became concerned with the possibility of overfortification of food. One company was pushing highly fortified cane sugar. The FDA thought sugar was an inappropriate vehicle for fortification because it might encourage excess sugar intake. The FDA lost the battle on this case but soon convened formal hearings to arrive at nutritionally sound fortification laws.[2]

The prudent approach of the FDA was effectively derailed by the mad rush to solve the malnutrition problem in the late 1960s and early 1970s. The highly misinterpreted Ten State Nutrition Survey and the political maneuverings of liberal Democrats pushed nutritionists into the limelight at the White House Conference on Food, Nutrition and Health, which was held in December 1969. To stem the perceived epidemic of iron deficiency, the nutritionists recommended that the level of iron enrichment be raised.[1-3]

Then big business got into the act. To maintain their products as the chief vehicles for fortification, and to increase the nutritional selling points, the American Bakers Association and the Millers National Federation made a formal proposal to the FDA to *quadruple* the amount of iron in wheat flour and bakery products.[2,3] In competition with meat products and other good sources of iron, the grain industry saw an opportunity to increase their market share at the neighborhood grocery store.

More Iron for the People

The FDA had a short memory. Abandoning its cautious approach, it responded to the political and industrial pressures by issuing its own recommendation, published April 1, 1970, in the *Federal Register*, to *triple* the quantity of iron in these foodstuffs.[4] This brought a firestorm of protest in public hearings, largely from concerned physicians led by Dr. Margaret A. Krikker, a general practitioner whose husband had iron overload, and by hematologist and iron expert Dr. William Crosby. By one count, only sixteen physicians endorsed the proposal as against 174 who opposed it.[3]

Lacking the political clout of industrial groups and the American Medical Association, the 174 physicians had only science on their side; they also did not have any financial incentives for their actions. Their objections fell into two general categories.

First, this less vocal faction of scientists had always had serious doubts about the "epidemic" of iron deficiency in America. Many of them, in stark disagreement with established "experts," did not believe in the classification of a disease purely on the basis of blood tests with no regard for symptoms or lack thereof. Furthermore, the truly anemic individual often has a bleeding problem, and early detection could save his or her life. The masking of this symptom by oversupplementation with iron only delays the diagnosis. True anemia is a serious medical condition, and the patient should be in experienced hands. As one physician put it, "The anemic woman should be going to the doctor, not the grocer." In the minds of these 174 physicians, fortification of foods for everyone in the population is an inefficient, scattershot approach to a serious medical problem that affects only a few individuals.[3,5,6]

Second, the most important reason for not artificially increasing the levels of iron in foods is that it may be dangerous for those individuals who consume a lot of those foods or for individuals who have an inherited condition that leads to iron overload (see Chapter 7). If the FDA fortification measure were to be adopted, it was estimated that a substantial fraction of young men would be getting *ten times* their RDA of iron every day—a level that has been shown to lead to heart and liver problems and even death. For those individuals who simply absorb too much iron, the risk is even greater. The question was easy for the 174 physicians to ask: why risk the health of the general population to help a few who should be under a doctor's care anyway?[5,7]

Drs. Krikker and Crosby have also pointed out that not only is iron fortification dangerous, it is illegal![5,8] The Delaney Amendment, a 1958 measure introduced by a New York congressman, James Delaney, specifically prohibits food companies from using additives that cause cancer in laboratory animals. Excess iron is known to cause liver cancer in both animals and humans. The fact that iron is a natural nutrient with important uses in the body should not blind us in our quest for utmost safety. Cholesterol has the same characteristics, but no one would propose to add more cholesterol to foods to solve a deficiency problem suffered by a few individuals.

Those physicians opposed to fortification thought they were victorious in 1977–1978 when the FDA commissioner, Donald Kennedy, who clearly saw the problems, struck down the proposal. In the *Federal Register* of August 29, 1978, Commissioner Kennedy wrote:[4]

> There is insufficient evidence that the augmentation in iron-fortified bread would ameliorate the condition of those who need iron. . . .
> There are no adequate studies showing the safety of the increased levels of iron in bread. . . . Therefore the proponents of augmentation have failed to sustain their burden of proof. . . .

Because of the findings and conclusions above, the aug-
mentation of iron-fortification of bread . . . should not be
approved.

Remarkably, with no new data in hand, some lower-level FDA
bureaucrats went ahead in 1979 and mandated a 50 percent
increase in the iron content in flour.[4] This halfway measure was
largely a response to pressures from industry groups, like the
American Bakers Association and the Pennwalt Corporation, a
major supplier of vitamin-iron enrichment premixes for the milling industry. The opponents of fortification were appalled by
this kowtowing to industry pressures and the lack of regard for
the previous commissioner's recommendations. The 174 physicians could now clearly see how difficult it would be to get
America iron-balanced.

Iron Pills

The debate surrounding iron fortification of flour was so fierce
partly because most people would be unknowingly increasing
their iron loads by eating widely available products made from
enriched flour. An equally important trend, however, has been
the *voluntary* consumption of iron pills or tonics, multivitamin-
mineral supplements, and highly fortified "supplement foods."

The vitamin supplement industry received an important boost
when in 1976 Senator William Proxmire performed a little leg-
islative sleight-of-hand to free up the industry from many federal
constraints.[9] The FDA was moving to classify excess doses of
vitamins as drugs, requiring ample—and expensive—evidence
that the health benefits are indeed produced. Vitamin manufacturers and the health food industry vigorously opposed this
attempt to regulate "natural" substances.

In the end, the Senate ratified the Proxmire amendment in
order to preserve the consumer's freedom of choice in the vitamin market. The bill allows *no* limit to be set on

the potency, number, combination, amount or variety of any synthetic or natural vitamin, mineral, or other substance or ingredient unless the amount recommended to be consumed is injurious to health.

Manufacturers were elated, of course. A vice president of the J. B. Williams Company, the makers of Geritol, proclaimed, "A number of major products, including Geritol, will no longer be forced to change formulation to comply with a government recipe based on FDA's version of what is rational." Soon you could buy vitamin tablets in amounts up to 33,000 percent of the U.S. RDA! The FDA commissioner at the time, Dr. Alexander Schmidt, lamented, "It opens up the field to fraud. Somebody could bottle sawdust and sell it as a food supplement."[9,10]

The vitamin-mineral supplement industry, which began in the health food store but has long since arrived at the grocery store, has grown into a $3-billion-a-year business. It is estimated that 40 percent of the U.S. population takes some form of vitamin or mineral supplement without a prescription.[11,12]

Iron supplements, either alone or in the multivitamin-multimineral "stress pills," are a significant fraction of this market. Though people usually know they are increasing their iron intake, few know of the potential dangers. They have heard that large amounts of vitamin C, for example, may be good for them, and at worst will simply lead to "expensive urine." But such is not the case with iron, since there is no efficient exit route. Chronic iron supplementation will increase the body's burden of excess iron and, as discussed in Parts 3 and 4, can lead to serious health consequences.

The worst offenders in the iron supplementation market are shown in the table below. A more complete list of the iron content in supplements is given in Appendix C.

**Selected Iron and Multivitamin-Mineral Supplements[a]
Containing High Amounts of Iron Per Recommended Dose[13]**

		IRON CONTENT	
Product Name	*Company Name*	*milligrams*	*% RDA[b]*
Hytinic capsules	Hyrex	150	833%
Niferex capsules	Central	150	833%
Vitron-C Plus	Fisons	132	733%
Ferancee-HP	Stuart	110	611%
Fumaral spancaps	Vortech	108	600%
Fero-Grad-500 tablets	Abbott	105	583%
Fero-Gradumet tablets	Abbott	105	583%
Generet-500 tablets	Goldline	105	583%
Iberet filmtabs	Abbott	105	583%
Iberet-500 filmtabs	Abbott	105	583%
Iberol filmtabs	Abbott	105	583%
Peritinic tablets	Lederle	100	556%
Rogenic	Forest	100	556%
Stuartinic tablets	Stuart	100	556%
Zentinic Pulvule capsules	Lilly	100	556%
Incremin with Iron syrup	Lederle	90 (15 milliliters)	500%

		IRON CONTENT	
Product Name	*Company Name*	*milligrams*	*% RDA*[b]
Secran/Fe elixir	Scherer	90 (15 milliliters)	500%
Iberet-Liquid	Abbott	78.75 (15 milliliters)	438%
Iberet-500 Liquid	Abbott	78.75 (15 milliliters)	438%
Ferancee	Stuart	67	372%
Vitron-C	Fisons	66	367%
Feosol tablets	SmithKline	65	361%
Fer-In-Sol capsules	Mead Johnson	60	333%
NeoVadrin Prenatal tablets	Mission	60	333%
Norlac tablets	Reid-Rowell	60	333%
Prenatal with Folic Acid tablets	Geneva Generics	60	333%
Prenavite tablets	Rugby	60	333%
Stuart Prenatal tablets	Stuart	60	333%
Zentron liquid	Lilly	60 (15 milliliters)	333%
Fergon Plus caplets	Winthrop	58	322%
Chel-Iron liquid	Kinney	50 (5 milliliters)	278%
Feosol capsules	SmithKline	50	278%
Ferralyn lanacaps	Lannett	50	278%

| | | IRON CONTENT | |
Product Name	Company Name	milligrams	% RDA[b]
Ferra-TD capsules	Goldline	50	278%
Ferro-Dok TR capsules	Major	50	278%
Ferro-Sequels	Lederle	50	278%
Ferrous-S.Q.L. capsules	Goldline	50	278%
Geriamic tablets	Vortech	50	278%
Geriot tablets	Goldline	50	278%
Geritol Complete tablets	SmithKline Beecham	50	278%
Geritol liquid	SmithKline Beecham	50 (15 milliliters)	278%
Niferex tablets	Central	50	278%
Niferex with Vitamin C tablets	Central	50	278%
Slow Fe tablets	Ciba	50	278%
Cal-Prenal Improved tablets	Vortech	49.3	274%
Fumaral elixir	Vortech	45 (1 milliliter)	250%
Natalins tablets	Mead Johnson	45	250%
Feosol elixir	SmithKline	44 (5 milliliters)	244%
Chel-Iron tablets	Kinney	40	222%

Product Name	Company Name	IRON CONTENT milligrams	% RDA[b]
Fermalox tablets	Rorer	40	222%
Mol-Iron tablets	Schering	39	217%
Mol-Iron with Vitamin C	Schering	39	217%

[a]Excludes prescription supplements for pregnant women.
[b]Based on the current U.S. RDA for iron of 18 milligrams.

Supercereals

In addition to pills and tonics, excess iron is also contained in heavily supplemented foods. The most pervasive of these are the supplement cereals like Total and Product 19, which have combined sales in excess of $150 million per year. These types of products are an important part of the powerful $7 billion breakfast cereal business.[14-17] The main selling point is that each serving contains 100 percent of the RDA for vitamins and minerals. That column of 100s in the nutritional table on the side of the box, as well as the commercials comparing "one bowl of Total" to several bowls of regular cereal, lead consumers to think that if they just eat that one bowl they are set for the day. But what about the excessive accumulation of potentially harmful nutrients like iron? Since the RDAs are generally set higher than people's actual requirements, iron accumulation is a real possibility for those individuals who consume the products over long periods or have inherited disorders such as iron-overload disease (hemochromatosis).

Since the 100-percents are a critical selling point for these products, manufacturers adjust the amounts of different nutrients in response to changes in the nation's standards. This can lead to excessive amounts of some nutrients, such as iron. For example, Total cereal, first introduced by General Mills in 1961, originally contained 100 percent of the Minimum Daily

Requirement (MDR) of iron and vitamins. When the nation shifted from MDRs to the more liberal RDAs in 1974, the company increased the amounts of the nutrients two to six times their original level to keep those valuable 100-percents.[17] This increased the iron content of one serving of Total from 10 to 18 milligrams. Because the adult RDAs are usually set at the highest amount required by certain groups, the value used for iron is really that for menstruating women and is clearly excessive for men and older women, whose RDAs are 10 milligrams. Since people are absorbing iron from other foods as well, the excess iron in these supercereals is going to add to the iron burden in the liver and other organs.

Here is a short list of popular cereals and their iron content. Note how many of them have added iron.

Iron Content Per Serving of Selected Breakfast Cereals (U.S. Market)

Product Name	Company Name	IRON CONTENT[a] milligrams	% RDA[b]
*Total	General Mills	18	100%
*Product 19	Kellogg's	18	100%
*Just Right	Kellogg's	18	100%
*Raisin Bran	Kellogg's	18	100%
*Cheerios	General Mills	8.1	45%
*Grape-Nuts	General Foods	8.1	45%
*Grape-Nuts Flakes	General Foods	8.1	45%
*Bran Flakes	General Foods	8.1	45%
*Oat Flakes	General Foods	8.1	45%
*Natural Raisin Bran	General Foods	6.3	35%
*Fruit and Fibre	General Foods	5.4–6.3	30–35%
*Quaker Oat Bran	Quaker Oats	5.4	30%
*Wheaties	General Mills	4.5	25%
*Cocoa Puffs	General Mills	4.5	25%
*All-Bran	Kellogg's	4.5	25%
*Oatbake	Kellogg's	4.5	25%
*Special K	Kellogg's	4.5	25%

Product Name	Company Name	IRON CONTENT[a] milligrams	% RDA[b]
*Mueslix	Kellogg's	4.5	25%
100% Bran	Nabisco	2.7	15%
*Rice Krispies	Kellogg's	1.8	10%
*Cracklin Oat Bran	Kellogg's	1.8	10%
*Crispix	Kellogg's	1.8	10%
*Frosted Flakes	Kellogg's	1.8	10%
*Corn Flakes	Kellogg's	1.8	10%
Shredded Wheat	Nabisco	0.72	4%
NutriGrain	Kellogg's	0.72	4%
Quaker 100% Natural	Quaker Oats	0.72	4%

[a]Asterisks denote cereals with added iron.
[b]Based on the current U.S. RDA for iron of 18 milligrams.

These cereals are likely to remain popular for some time because of their convenience and the nation's growing awareness of nutritional needs. The products are highly profitable for manufacturers since they command premium prices with very little added costs in the manufacturing process. Total, for example, is basically Wheaties coated with a cheap (two cents per box[18]) vitamin spray, but it sells for approximately eighty cents more per twelve-ounce box at the grocery store (in the Boston, Massachusetts, area). And, as you know, there is ample advertising for these products; the Kellogg's advertising budget in 1988, for example, was $683 million.[14]

The amount of iron in these cereals and other highly fortified foods will probably decrease somewhat as a result of the decrease in the RDA for premenopausal women in the 1989 version of the RDAs from 18 to 15 milligrams. This change will not take effect until 1992, when the U.S. RDAs that appear on food labels will be replaced with Reference Daily Intake (RDI) values. When this occurs, the U.S. RDI for iron will be 15 milligrams, and consequently the cereal companies will be adding 3 milligrams less iron to each serving of their products.

Fifteen milligrams of iron in one meal is still too much for most of us. It would be much better if excess iron were excluded from these cereals. (I cannot see that this would affect the sales: the products would still provide 100 percent of the RDA for all those important vitamins.) This approach would be much safer for the millions of people at risk for iron overload.

Fortification Today

The iron fortification battleground is somewhat silent today, though each side stands by its original views. The deregulation era of the Reagan and Bush administrations has done little to encourage a reexamination of fortification policy. If anything, the relationship between the FDA and industry has become even more cozy, with bureaucrats now being charged for taking bribes from companies such as those in the generic drug business.

In the flour and cereal business, it seems that the FDA has altered its once cautious views to more closely fit the deregulation atmosphere and industry's concerns. At a 1982 meeting of the Council on Fortification of the American Association of Cereal Chemists, a strong profortification group, the associate director for nutrition and food science of the FDA, Dr. Allan Forbes, opened his talk with comforting words to the industry group: "I am, and have been for a long time, an advocate of the rational addition of nutrients to foods."[2] In referring to a 1980 FDA action to free up restrictions on fortification, he added:

> In the interim period, nothing has happened to change this policy. If anything, it has been strengthened under the [Reagan] administration because it is fundamentally voluntary and serves as our basic guide to industry in the practice of modern rational nutrition science.

Later in the conference, a lawyer from the prestigious Washington law firm Covington and Burling, the one that successfully jousted with the Federal Trade Commission on behalf of the Geritol people, explained that the food industry had "misunderstood" the FDA's original decision to restrict excessive iron fortification of flour; the decision was a very close one, he said, and the FDA would happily reconsider it if more evidence in support of higher fortification was forthcoming. In the meantime, he added, industry had nothing to fear: "Unduly restrictive regulatory approaches to fortification by FDA have now been abandoned and are unlikely to return unless unwarranted fortification becomes prevalent in the future."

With this antiregulatory atmosphere, the burden of proof in the fortification controversy has really fallen on the concerned opponents, who must somehow provide irrefutable evidence that large-scale iron fortification has done more harm than good. In a medical environment that continues to emphasize the diagnosis and treatment of iron deficiency over that of iron overload, this is a very difficult, if not impossible, task. As I discuss in the following chapter, the early detection of hereditary iron overload (hemochromatosis) is quite low in this country: victims are often misdiagnosed for years. If we do not even know who these people are, how can we adequately study the effects of fortification on their health? In addition, the potential role of iron in widespread diseases like heart disease and cancer is just now surfacing and is not widely known. Without some shift in the medical establishment's view of iron, it is doubtful whether the safety of iron fortification in the U.S. will ever be adequately addressed.

Many interested physicians believe that an extensive study of the Swedish population may shed some light on the safety of iron fortification. For over forty years, the Swedes have consumed highly fortified flour (containing three times the iron of U.S. flour) and, as a result, their average daily intake of iron exceeds that of most other countries. Roughly 42 percent of the Swedish daily iron intake is from fortification iron, compared to about 25 percent in the U.S.[19]

A report in 1978 showed that Swedish men did appear to suffer from severe iron overload to a larger extent than other populations.[20] Five percent of the 200 men examined had high serum iron readings, with roughly 2.5 percent showing clear signs of iron overload. To date, it has not been determined whether iron fortification of flour is fully or even partly responsible for the apparent prevalence of this disease among Swedish men.

Some Swedish physicians continue to be concerned about their country's high level of iron fortification. Iron experts from around the world are often invited to Sweden to express their views on whether ill-effects may ensue. Unfortunately, many of these experts return home feeling that the Swedish fortification debate is often dominated by entrenched business interests—those companies producing iron supplements and iron-fortified foods—rather than the scientific issues.

Warning: Iron May Be Hazardous to Your Health

The scientists and consumers who are against excessive iron fortification of flour and cereals are hoping that, at the very least, the FDA will add some warning labels on products that might be hazardous to those who have the potential for iron overload. (Once again, this will of course not help the hundreds of thousands of people in this country who are unaware they have the disease.)

The Iron Overload Diseases Association, based in North Palm Beach, Florida, is currently "educating" the FDA and relevant industries on this matter. In a recent newsletter, the organization published an excerpt of their correspondence with the FDA:[21]

> The members of the Iron Overload Diseases Association in all of our 50 states make it constantly clear that they want to find breakfast cereals and other foods that do NOT have added iron.
>
> When iron is added, our members want a caution notice: "Warning—This product contains an iron additive and should not be used by anyone who is iron overloaded."
>
> Families who have lost a hemochromatosis patient . . . take bitter notice that the patient unknowingly ingested iron-laden food.

It is amazing that these measures have not been taken sooner. The situation with iron labeling for hemochromatosis patients is exactly analogous to that with aspartame (Nutrasweet) labeling for those with phenylketonuria, a liver enzyme deficiency. Yet the latter condition affects only very small numbers of people, while hemochromatosis strikes over one million in the U.S. alone.

While the Iron Overload Diseases Association faces an uphill battle in their labeling efforts due to ingrained notions about the safety of iron, they are making some progress. One company, the Mead Johnson division of Bristol-Myers Squibb, has recently added the label "Not to be taken by individuals with hemochromatosis" to their vitamin-iron supplements used in pregnancy.

To understand the energy behind this movement to carefully label products for hemochromatosis patients and to increase awareness of this disease, you have to meet some of its victims. In the following chapter, you'll learn about John Mury, Roberta Crawford, and others who have suffered from iron overload.

Part 3

VICTIMS OF IRON OVERLOAD: MAKE SURE YOU ARE NOT AMONG THEM

7

Hereditary Iron-Overload Disease: A Hidden Killer

Hemochromatosis, an inherited iron-overloading disease, lurks among us. When you are sitting in an airplane, movie theater, or some other public place, look around you: chances are that at least one of the people present has the full-blown form of hemochromatosis. In this deadly disease, abnormally high levels of iron are absorbed from the diet, and the excess metal deposits in several organs within the body. The dire consequences include heart disease, liver cancer, diabetes, impotence, and even death. Unfortunately, even with today's advanced health care, many hemochromatosis victims go undetected for years, accumulating higher and higher levels of toxic iron.

There is also a less severe form of hemochromatosis which affects even more people. On average, there might be about twenty to thirty of these individuals in the airplane or theater with you. (Note that this group is more likely to include you!) These individuals are also likely to absorb more iron from their diet than they require, though doctors are still debating whether they suffer any tissue damage or predisposition for other diseases. What is most important for people with this form of hemochromatosis is that they can pass on the disease to their children, and if they happen to have children with someone who also has the disease, the children can acquire the more deadly, full-blown version.

Hemochromatosis is one of the most common inherited diseases. More people in the U.S. are affected by this disease than cystic fibrosis, Huntington's disease, and muscular dystrophy combined. But you won't hear of any celebrities raising funds to combat iron overload: no twenty-four-hour telethons, no government programs to increase awareness, no huge foundations with millions of dollars to spend on research and education. Hemochromatosis is the forgotten disease: it lurks insidiously in our society, hidden both from patients and, unfortunately, many doctors.

Victims and their families wonder how many lives have to be lost before the word gets out. How much suffering and debilitation will unknowing victims have to endure? How many more million-dollar lawsuits have to be filed?

The urgent need these people feel for increasing the awareness of this disease stems in part from the fact that, unlike many inherited diseases, there is a good treatment for hemochromatosis: regular withdrawal of the high-iron blood draws the toxic metal out of the tissues, preventing further damage. Many years of life—and even apparently total cures—can be achieved if the disease is caught early enough. But it usually is not.

This is the true story of men, women, and "rust." With hemochromatosis, people can accumulate ten to fifty grams of iron in their bodies, enough to set off metal detectors in airports. These victims are the clearest examples of the deleterious effects of excess iron in the human body. Their stories here are the black-and-white proof that iron can kill.

John and Hedwig Mury

Hedwig Mury remembers her husband John fondly. In her native German accent, she told me over and over what a "wonderful, wonderful man" he was. Through their twenty-three years of marriage, until John passed away in 1990, they hardly ever argued. If she was upset about something, John would just hug her and ask her softly what the problem was. He was "such a good and gentle man."

John had hemochromatosis, and his story is sadly typical of many people with this disease. He was misdiagnosed for years and then struggled to keep the damage that had been done to his body from killing him. The disease and its mishandling by doctors robbed the Murys of many pleasures in life. Profound fatigue followed by liver and heart disease, arthritis, impotence, and diabetes all took their toll on John and, indirectly, on Hedwig.

John's first symptom, experienced in his early forties, was profound fatigue. He later said that he felt "washed out and tired all the time." When he was forty-five, a black stool indicated that he had internal bleeding. In trying to find out what was wrong with John, the doctors went so far as to perform a liver biopsy, in which a small piece of liver is taken and analyzed under a microscope. In John's case, unfortunately, the sample was not examined closely enough. While the doctors did detect cirrhosis, the hardening of the liver with fibrous scar tissue often caused by excess alcohol, they failed to notice its true cause: huge deposits of iron. It should be pointed out that John was a very light drinker.

John's condition began to deteriorate in a pattern typical of hemochromatosis. He gradually got arthritis, but no one thought that this was related to his liver problem. Besides, he later said that "you sort of get used to arthritis."

Then, at age fifty-one, John had his first attack of angina, the sharp chest pain that signals heart disease. John was told that a coronary bypass operation might solve his heart trouble as well as his fatigue, so he submitted to the operation. But it did nothing to relieve his "washed-out" feeling. In addition, a cardiologist actually gave him iron supplements that were supposed to help him recover from the operation. In John's case, this only increased the amount of iron accumulating in his body.

Then in 1981 a hematologist diagnosed John's sister Alice as having hemochromatosis. She was experiencing symptoms similar to John's, though doctors thought that her problems might be due to drinking. Alice and her family knew that alcohol was not the problem, and through persistence and the counsel of a good specialist they eventually located the cause.

John and his wife were visiting Alice's family when she came home from her first blood-withdrawal treatment (*phlebotomy*) to remove the excess iron. Everyone noticed that, in addition to their similar medical histories, they both had the bronzed, tan skin that is often present in hemochromatosis victims. (The excess iron somehow boosts the production of melanin, the tanning pigment.) John also had brown spots behind the nails on his fingers and toes. Alice had been alerted by her hematologist to look for affected family members. John was a clear possibility.

When John finally got the clear proof that hemochromatosis had indeed been his problem all along, he and his wife were shocked. Though he began the rigorous phlebotomy schedule immediately, to remove the toxic iron, they knew a great deal of damage had already been done to his body. Ten years of mishandling by doctors had caused great pain and anguish, in addition to lost income and huge medical bills.

In what is believed to be the first medical malpractice case in the U.S. focused on the failure to diagnose hemochromatosis, John and Hedwig Mury sued a total of five doctors, two of whom failed to see the iron deposits in the liver biopsy taken in 1972. It was a bitter lawsuit; Hedwig says now that the whole process nearly drove her crazy. Her husband was questioned for eight hours at one point by five aggressive lawyers. They harassed him, accusing him of being a heavy drinker. Hedwig was questioned for two hours. She noted that they never bothered to ask her how it felt to see her husband sick and impotent.

Fortunately, the Murys located an expert on hemochromatosis who outclassed the other doctors and set the record straight. Hedwig now says that "he made mincemeat out of them—they were so scared! He gave them the lesson of their lives!" At this point, the doctors could see that their case was weak, and they settled out of court with the Murys for the substantial sum of half a million dollars.

Did the money mean much to the Murys? Not at all: they would have exchanged it at any point during the fiasco for John's good health. But they hoped that the award would send a few shock waves through the medical community and help doctors focus on the early detection of hemochromatosis.

John eventually died in 1990 at the age of sixty-three. He had stuck to the difficult treatment regimen: two years of weekly bleedings and then one every four to six weeks. But a great deal of damage had been done. In addition to his serious heart condition, diabetes had entered the picture. The phlebotomies probably extended his life, but not as much as they could have if he had been diagnosed in 1972 instead of nine years later. (John's sister Alice, two years younger than him, was not as badly affected and continues to do fine.)

The Bronze Man of Iron

Hemochromatosis is an enigmatic disease that has presented a formidable challenge to the medical community for ages. Dr. William Crosby, director of hematology at the Chapman Cancer Center in Joplin, Missouri, has called hemochromatosis a "constellation of diseases." It disguises itself in different combinations of somewhat common diseases, such as diabetes and liver and heart disease, and continues to fool even today's doctors.

The French were the first to pick out and describe hemochromatosis as a unique disorder.[1-3] In a clinical lecture published in 1865, Armand Trousseau, one of the great masters of medicine in France, described a case of a young man with diabetes and liver cirrhosis who also had an additional peculiar symptom: "From the time this man came into the hospital, I was struck by the almost bronzed appearance of his countenance."[1]

Soon thereafter a more complete picture of what we now know to be hemochromatosis was described by another French physician, Troisier, at a meeting of the Anatomical Society of Paris:[1]

> There was, in this [diabetic] patient, a brownish coloration of the skin of the face, of the neck and upper part of the chest, of the external genitalia, of the [groin], of the hands and forearms. This coloration was not uniform.
>
> In the places mentioned, there were irregularly rounded,

flat spots of a more pronounced brownish tint and islets of black pigment. The rest of the skin (trunk, abdomen, and extremities) had an ashen color. At the level of the right elbow there was a brownish placque.

The patient said that he had always been of sun-tanned color, but he believed that the brown color of his skin had become much more pronounced in the past two or three months.

He died [completely wasted away].

It is likely that this patient was described at a relatively advanced stage of the disease. Like John Mury, he had the suntanned skin and brown spots characteristic of hemochromatosis. But the "ashen color" spotted by Troisier indicates that, in addition to the excess production of melanin, the pigment that tans the skin, this patient had significant amounts of iron deposited directly in the skin. This causes the whitish-gray coloration.

Another important observation Troisier made was that, at autopsy, the liver and pancreas had an odd "rusty" coloration. In 1889, the German physician H. von Recklinghausen was the first to make the connection between this color and iron deposition. He identified certain iron-containing substances in the tissues of a cirrhosis patient. It was also von Recklinghausen who coined the term hemochromatosis (*hemo* = blood; *chroma* = color; *osis* = condition). He thought the rusty color of the tissues was caused by the breakdown of blood cells and capillaries, with subsequent deposition of iron-containing blood pigments.[1,2]

A number of other explanations for the disease were offered by the experts of the day. The French stuck to the original observation of their countrymen, maintaining that hemochromatosis was a particular form of diabetes referred to as "bronze diabetes." Other doctors thought it was primarily a liver disease with diabetic complications, perhaps stemming from excessive alcohol ingestion. But it was J. H. Sheldon, a British physician, who first suggested in 1927 that the iron deposition in hemochromatosis was caused by an inherited disorder in iron metabolism:[1]

The time taken for these deposits to accumulate is very long, and it is possible that the disease is an inborn error of metabolism, the accumulation being so slow that the characteristic clinical symptoms do not appear till middle age is reached.

At that time, Sheldon had no evidence that hemochromatosis ran in families, but the next year a case of two brothers was described that seemed to fit his hypothesis. Over the next eight years, Sheldon collected 365 cases of hemochromatosis from the world's medical literature, citing fourteen examples where the disease seemed to strike in two or more members of the same family. A new genetic disease had been discovered.

The Genetic Card Game

At the opening of this chapter, I mentioned that there are two major forms of hemochromatosis: a deadly, full-blown form of the disease, which was spotted by the nineteenth-century European physicians, and a more prevalent mild form. To understand the difference between these forms and to see how children inherit hemochromatosis, you have to know a little about the genetic card game, the ultimate "game of life."

We are all products of our genes, the packets of chemical information in each of our cells that determine our eye and hair color, our height, and other traits. Each gene is like a recipe card, telling the cell which substance to make, and how much.

We have two "decks" of these recipe cards: one from each of our parents. When a couple has a child, the decks are essentially shuffled and the child inherits a fresh set of cards composed of those from his parents. Though the combination that the child receives is unique, this individuality comes not from any new genes but from the shuffling of the more than 100,000 genes from each of the parents.

If one or both of the parents has a faulty gene, a card with a torn corner, it is likely that the child will too. Like a bad recipe that never seems to work, a faulty gene produces substances that do not fulfill their appointed tasks in the body. In the case of hemochromatosis, the bad gene is not identified, but it must have something to do with the handling of iron in the body.

Let us look at the most common inheritance pattern leading to hemochromatosis. If both parents carry a single copy of the bad gene for the disease (this is the mild form), then the children will fall into one of three categories.

First, there is a 25 percent chance that the child will be "dealt a bad hand" and inherit two copies of the bad recipe card. The child is said to be *homozygous*, "of the same egg," with respect to the hemochromatosis gene. Since two copies of any gene are all a person gets, the child will be left without the proper chemical instructions for making some important component of his or her iron metabolism machinery. This is the full-blown form of the disease.

There is a 50 percent chance that the child will inherit only one copy of the bad gene for hemochromatosis, not two. This is known as the *heterozygous* state of the disease—that is, "of different eggs"—and is the mild form of hemochromatosis. We also say that the child is a "carrier" of the disease, since he or she has the potential to pass on the bad gene to further generations. Since heterozygotes still possess one good copy of the gene, their body cells can manufacture the key component of iron metabolism machinery that homozygotes cannot. Nonetheless, in the case of hemochromatosis, heterozygotes may still exhibit some differences in iron metabolism in comparison to the general population. The possible health effects are discussed later in this chapter.

Finally, there is also a 25 percent chance that the child will be "dealt a pair of aces" and inherit only the good genes from each of the parents. This child would not have hemochromatosis and would not pass on any tendency for the disease to following generations.

So you can see that two parents who are both unknowingly heterozygotes for hemochromatosis can produce a homozygous child who will most likely become iron-overloaded during his or her lifetime. There is also the possibility that a homozygote will mate with a heterozygote. In this case, there is even a greater chance—50 percent—that the resulting child will be homozygous. Though this should not happen too often, due to the odds against two such people having children together, there are cases where hemochromatosis has been seen to run in a family for two, three, and possibly four generations.

How Many People Have the Full-Blown Form of Hemochromatosis?

It is unfortunate that hemochromatosis has long been considered by doctors to be a very rare disease. As a result, millions of people in the world have died from it unknowingly. Part of the problem has been that many victims do not exhibit the "classic triad" of symptoms—liver disease, diabetes, and bronze or grayish skin—that was described by early researchers. In John Mury's case, for example, diabetes was a relatively late manifestation of the disease. In addition, his skin color took on a bronze tint over a long period of time, and so this was not caught by his doctors. Many victims who do suffer from the classic triad do so only in the more advanced stages of the disease.

The notion that hemochromatosis is rare has been imbedded in medical textbooks for years. Each new class of doctors would read that only one in 20,000 people—around 10,000 people in the U.S.—has hemochromatosis, and almost all of those affected by it are men. But these estimates were based on fairly old studies using very insensitive diagnostic criteria.

The latest studies show that hemochromatosis is a great deal more common than previously thought. The most important of these studies has been that of Dr. Corwin Edwards and colleagues at the University of Utah School of Medicine. In a 1988 *New England Journal of Medicine* article, they reported the results of an analysis of blood samples from 11,065 presumably healthy donors.[4] Using a relatively simple technique, they measured the extent to which transferrin, the iron-carrying "wheelbarrow" protein in the blood, was saturated with iron. People with hemochromatosis absorb too much iron, and their transferrin molecules become almost filled. The most sensitive and accurate diagnostic criterion for homozygous hemochromatosis turned out to be a transferrin saturation value of 62 percent or more— that is, 62 percent or more of the iron-carrying capacity of the blood is used up. One out of every 200 donors was found to have the disease by this criterion. This estimate is a *hundred times* more than that printed in many medical textbooks!

These results have now placed hemochromatosis near the top of the list of purely inherited disorders and diseases in which inherited factors play an important role. As you can see in the table below, hemochromatosis, affecting approximately five per thousand individuals, ranks third in this list, following closely behind various disorders of fat (or cholesterol) metabolism (which lead to increased risk of heart attacks), and diabetes. In the U.S. alone, over one million people are expected to have the full-blown, homozygous form of hemochromatosis. As Dr. Virgil Fairbanks, a hemochromatosis expert at the Mayo Clinic, has said, "The affliction is epidemic."

Unlike many genetic diseases, hemochromatosis seems to affect many different ethnic groups. A 1988 survey of U.S. hemochromatosis patients conducted by the Iron Overload Diseases Association found that no particular group was spared. Twenty-three different national origins and four races were represented in rough proportion to their fraction of the U.S. population.[6]

Estimated Frequency of Various Genetic Diseases[5]

Disease	Frequency Per 100,000 People
Disorders of fat metabolism (all forms)	at least 1200
Diabetes (all forms)	1000
HEREDITARY HEMOCHROMATOSIS	500
Primary gout	200
Down's syndrome	170
Sickle-cell anemia (U.S. blacks)	150
Klinefelter's syndrome (males)	140
XYY syndrome (males)	130

Disease	Frequency Per 100,000 People
Triple X syndrome (females)	at least 100
Adult polycystic kidney disease	80
Turner's syndrome (females)	67
Cystic fibrosis	40
Huntington's disease	40
Muscular dystrophy (males)	14
Phenylketonuria	8

What Are the Odds That You Have the Mild Form of Hemochromatosis?

Just as it is easier in a game of poker to get a single ace rather than a pair, the odds of inheriting only one bad hemochromatosis gene are much greater than the odds of getting two. Genetic experts have estimated that about 13.4 percent of the U.S. population—one out of seven people—is heterozygous for hemochromatosis: that is over thirty million people! Many scientists regard the hemochromatosis gene as one of the most common abnormal genes in the human species.[4]

Why would this be so? Wouldn't millions of years of evolution give those families without the defect a selective survival advantage? This is true for many genetic defects, but not for those like hemochromatosis that most often lead to deleterious health effects only *after* the major reproductive years. As long as each generation can successfully reproduce, there will be no advantage to those free of the hemochromatosis gene.

The widespread nature of the hemochromatosis gene also suggests that at one time it may have been advantageous for certain populations that had a difficult time getting enough iron in their diets. This may be especially true for women, who require more iron during pregnancy. Those with the extra iron-absorbing power of the hemochromatosis gene may have had a better chance of giving birth to healthy infants. Over time, this would have the effect of enriching the population with this particular gene.

In Western countries today, however, it is likely that the heterozygous state for hemochromatosis can only do us harm, not good. Our diets are rich in iron, and few of us need to build up our already substantial reserves. Scientists have found that heterozygotes do have a tendency to absorb more iron than normal folks, though not nearly to the degree of their homozygous counterparts. As it turns out, the heterozygotes have iron levels that are often near the high end of the "normal" range. It has proved impossible to identify them through blood tests alone because of this considerable overlap.[7,8] Nonetheless, anyone with high iron levels, whether they possess the hemochromatosis gene or not, may be at higher risk for heart disease, cancer, and other diseases.

A Storage Tank With No Bottom

Now let us turn back to the full-blown (homozygous) form of hemochromatosis and get a closer look at how a single bad recipe card or gene leads to iron men and iron women. Scientists still have to figure out the details of this process, but many are leaning toward the following scenario.

Normally, the cells lining the intestine have an effective, though suicidal, way to prevent iron overload. These cells act like intermediate storage depots, temporarily sequestering incoming iron inside the spherical protein called ferritin. If the body needs more iron, the intestinal cells let some through. However, if we have enough, the entire cell, with its piles of ferritin iron, eventually sloughs off into the interior of the intestine and is excreted. This constant loss of iron-containing intestinal cells contributes significantly to the daily loss of iron. Without this mechanism, iron accumulation in the body is more likely.

A key step in this process is in the proper storage of the excess iron in the ferritin storage bins. Some scientists feel that the defect in hemochromatosis victims is on the recipe card that tells the intestinal cell how to manufacture its own ferritin. You can think of it this way: imagine that the hemochromatosis gene specifies the construction of ferritin storage bins with *no bottom.* The incoming iron falls right through and ends up floating around freely in the intestinal cell. Not restrained in its proper storage place, this free iron continually enters the body, leading to iron overload.

Iron Variability

The severity of iron overload in hemochromatosis victims varies widely. Some people acquire a few grams of iron, and some up to thirty grams. By the way, the stories of iron-loaded patients setting off metal detectors at airports are true. Dr. J. Robert Campbell of Tampa, Florida, a hemochromatosis victim himself, once rang the bells at the high-security system in Rome, Italy. He had to convince the guards that he was not a hijacker—just someone with a highly magnetic personality![6]

The amount of iron that builds up in hemochromatosis victims varies for many reasons, presumably due to complex factors including biological variation among individuals. One important factor that these people can control is, of course, their total iron intake. Someone who eats high-iron steaks all the time will obviously build up iron levels faster than a vegetarian. In fact, iron overload does not appear even to have been reported in countries like India, where diets are often inadequate, particularly with regard to iron.

Another variable that might contribute to the broad range of iron levels in hemochromatosis patients is the extent to which they drink alcoholic beverages. First, it is important to know that wines, particularly reds, have substantial iron content and have been thought to be responsible for some cases of iron overload. (More on this topic in Chapters 8 and 17.) In fact, some doctors believe that hemochromatosis was first spotted in France because of that country's propensity for red wine. Moreover, alcohol and iron overload are a dangerous combination because alcohol increases iron-absorption rates and excessive alcohol independently adds to the organ damage already present in iron-overload patients.

Signs and Symptoms

Just as the amounts of iron in hemochromatosis victims vary, so do the symptoms that eventually bring them into the doctor's office. It is possible that there are several versions of the disease but researchers simply have not been able to identify them.

Listed below are the most common symptoms of hemochromatosis. If you have two or more of them, ask your doctor to perform a full-scale blood-iron test (the transferrin saturation test) for this disease. See Chapter 20 for more information.

Following are the most common sites of iron overload and the diseases that result:[3,7,9]

The Liver. The liver receives a great deal of the excess iron in hemochromatosis and suffers considerable damage. You may remember that in John Mury's case, presented at the beginning of this chapter, it was liver disease that initially sent him into the hospital. Excess iron leads to the formation of scar tissue and eventually cirrhosis. The latter often leads to death in hemochromatosis patients. These individuals are also at considerable risk for liver cancer, a disease that is normally not that prevalent in Western societies. Researchers have estimated that for a hemochromatosis patient, the risk of dying from liver cancer is over two hundred times the normal rate.

Symptom	Frequency of Symptom in Hemochromatosis Patients[9]
Weakness, fatigue	83%
Abdominal pain	58%
Diabetes	55%
Arthritis	43%
Impotence (males)	38%
Amenorrhea (females)	22%
Shortness of breath	15%
Neurologic symptoms (disorientation, depression, hearing loss)	6%

The Heart. Complications involving the heart muscle are another common cause of death in hemochromatosis patients. Iron-induced tissue damage hinders the pumping ability of the heart, and it becomes enlarged. When the heart cannot pump enough blood, the body retains salt and water, and the blood volume increases. The excess fluid can back up into the lungs and other tissues. This form of heart disease, called *congestive cardiomyopathy*, leads to death in hemochromatosis patients about three hundred times more often than in the general population.

The Pancreas and Diabetes. Damage to the insulin-producing cells in the pancreas has long been thought to be an important cause of diabetes in hemochromatosis patients. However, the current view is that other effects of iron overload, such as liver damage, as well as a hereditary disposition for diabetes, may be responsible for the high rate of this disease in people who are iron-overloaded. Diabetes, which interferes with the proper burning of carbohydrates as fuels, is often responsible for some of the nonspecific symptoms, such as weakness or chronic fatigue.

The Joints. Arthritis, caused by the deposition of iron in the joints, is a common, early symptom of hemochromatosis. Stiffness in the joints of the fingers and hands and later in the knees, shoulders, and spine are common.

The Pituitary Gland and Infertility. Iron-induced damage to the brain's anterior pituitary gland causes greatly diminished secretion of the hormones necessary for sexual function. This often occurs in younger patients. Men become impotent, lose their libido, and may also experience breast enlargement and loss of body hair. Women lose their libido, have difficulty conceiving, and their periods may stop altogether.

An Ancient Treatment

The treatment of hemochromatosis is one that is right out of ancient medical lore: bloodletting. Removal of a pint of blood gets rid of about 200 milligrams of toxic iron. The bone marrow cells respond by speeding up the production of red blood cells and drawing more iron out of the liver and other overloaded tissues. Hemochromatosis patients who have accumulated ten to thirty grams of iron generally need one to three years of weekly phlebotomies to deplete their iron loads. After that, periodic phlebotomies every two to three months are sufficient to prevent the reaccumulation of iron.

It is a difficult schedule for many hemochromatosis victims. Though it is very safe and the pain is minimal, it is repetitive, somewhat time consuming, and the temporary anemia it creates can lead to fatigue. But most patients view the excess iron as a poison polluting their bodies, and they desperately want to get rid of it as fast as possible.

Over the years, many physicians challenged the idea that the iron was actually causing the damage in hemochromatosis, and they wondered whether it really had to be removed. Perhaps it was difficult for these physicians to abandon their rosy image of iron, the wonder mineral. They even thought that the benefits of phlebotomy treatments were purely psychological. In 1960, one noted physician wrote:[2]

> Practically all patients have an initial period when their sense of well-being and strength improves. The strong suggestive power of a blood-letting episode has been known for centuries, however, and the enthusiasm of the physician for such a program undoubtedly has an additive effect.

Still, most physicians thought that the iron must have something to do with the tissue damage and preferred to get rid of it.

A West German study, published in a 1985 issue of the *New England Journal of Medicine*, has provided the most convincing proof that phlebotomy works miracles for hemochromatosis.[9] Dr. Claus Niederau and his coworkers studied 163 hemochromatosis patients for an average of ten years. When phlebotomies were not instituted, it was known that the fraction of patients who survived for at least five years after their diagnosis was only about 18 percent; the ten-year survival rate was only 6 percent. The West German study found that hemochromatosis patients whose livers were not cirrhotic could have a normal life span if phlebotomies were instituted immediately upon diagnosis. Even if the disease had progressed to the cirrhotic stage, there was a 75 percent chance that they could survive ten years with the treatment.

The study also found that the removal of iron through phlebotomy improved heart conditions, removed the skin pigmentation, and for 50 to 70 percent of the patients, improved the functional capacity of the liver. Diabetic conditions and arthritis improved in some subjects. Unfortunately, the phlebotomies did not seem to reduce the chance of getting liver cancer or restore sexual function.

The overall safety and success of phlebotomy in the treatment of iron overload is the reason I have included it in the Iron Balance Health Plan. See Chapter 18 for more details.

Medical Bungling

Since there is a sound and effective treatment for hemochromatosis, you can understand the frustration that victims and their families feel when people go undiagnosed for years. One of these victims, Roberta Crawford, struggled for years with various symptoms including anemia, fatigue, and repeated respiratory infections before receiving her diagnosis. She has since founded the Iron Overload Diseases Association in North Palm Beach, Florida, the largest patient support and medical education group for hemochromatosis.

Mrs. Crawford, a former journalist, wrote of her experience in an article published in 1980 by *Good Housekeeping*.[10] This article marks the beginning of the association and a small but growing movement to make the public aware of iron's dark side. In it, she told of how she was shuttled from doctor to doctor with no end in sight. Several of the doctors even encouraged her to take iron, the very substance that was destroying her body. When she was finally diagnosed by a specialist as having iron overload, Roberta and her husband, Vern, were shocked.

> When I got home, I told Vern. "At last I have a diagnosis. I have hemochromatosis."
> He was horrified. "Is there a cure?" he asked.

"Yes, there's one treatment. . . . The doctors have to bleed me. They have to take away a pint of my blood every week from now on."

Neither of us knew what to say. We both thought of the decades I'd spent taking doctor-prescribed iron pills to cure my anemia, increase my hemoglobin, raise my red-cell count, and build up my blood. Now all that treatment for anemia was down the drain. . . .

The scariest thing . . . is that many doctors are not even aware they can kill their patients by prescribing too much iron. That's what almost happened to me. I hope this story keeps it from happening to others.

The tragic irony in Mrs. Crawford's story is that she was medicated with iron when, in fact, she needed the exact opposite: the removal of excess iron from her body. The popularity of anemia as a diagnosis and iron supplements as a cure-all for vague complaints, particularly in women, has done untold harm to thousands who are unaware that they are hemochromatosis victims, and perhaps to others as well. In a survey conducted by Mrs. Crawford's Iron Overload Diseases Association, it was found that up to 25 percent of hemochromatosis patients actually got iron supplements from their doctors at some point prior to their diagnosis.[6] Why don't doctors measure iron levels before prescribing iron? If they did, the percentage of hemochromatosis patients diagnosed would go up, and fewer people would be taking iron supplements unnecessarily.

Women and Hemochromatosis

The subject of the treatment of female hemochromatosis victims is an important issue to the Iron Overload Diseases Association. Not only did its founder, Mrs. Crawford, have trouble getting diagnosed, but thousands like her have shared this experience. Many doctors still believe that hemochromatosis affects men ten times more than women, since women lose iron through menstruation. But the amount of iron lost is often not enough to balance the enormous influx of the toxic metal. In addition, many younger patients fail to have regular periods. In fact, sometimes the cause of amenorrhea *is* hemochromatosis.

One recent case concerning hemochromatosis in a young woman was particularly tragic. At age seventeen she became amenorrheic, though her periods had been normal for the preceding five years. Over seven years, she was seen by six physicians, including gynecologists and endocrinologists. They diagnosed a hormonal abnormality but failed to notice the signs of liver damage that were evident in some of her blood tests. She then developed congestive cardiomyopathy, the heart condition that is common in hemochromatosis, and died at age twenty-four while awaiting a heart transplant.[11]

Another recent case has a better ending. Though it took many years, twenty-eight-year-old Jennifer Hyland was finally diagnosed as having hemochromatosis at a relatively young age; now her prognosis is excellent. She is concerned, however, about her ability to have children and is now seeing a fertility expert. She told her story in a recent edition of the Iron Overload Diseases Association's newsletter:[6]

> I should have been diagnosed at age 11 when tests showed high iron and [liver damage]. "Hemochromatosis" was mentioned on my chart. Unfortunately the doctor did not follow up. He was satisfied to call it hepatitis.
>
> The delay of 15 more years has caused me an immeasurable amount of heartache and pain.
>
> I was always one of the more athletic children in my neighborhood until the "hepatitis." Over the next 15 years my endurance steadily declined. I couldn't understand why I had turned into such a "lemon." Diets, exercise, nothing worked. I was always exhausted.
>
> In 1986 something happened that I couldn't figure out. My periods stopped. I was 24. The same thing had happened to my sister, Joyce, at age 28. Joyce had undergone years of declining health, too, and was then diagnosed with diabetes. Joyce's color was a dull greenish tone. We were all worried about her.
>
> Finally a doctor did test her [serum] ferritin and trans-

ferrin saturation. Diagnosis! At last! When the rest of the family was tested, my iron levels were twice as high as my older sister's! My ferritin was 4800 units. [This is over one hundred times the normal value for women Jennifer's age.]

I had a very hard time facing phlebotomies at first. Then I started thinking of the iron as poison. My schedule was two phlebotomies a week, 500–600 cubic centimeters. I could see that one or two phlebotomies a month would do nothing. . . .

I was determined to stick with it. I had to keep reminding myself there really was a light at the end of the tunnel. After a year and a half I was completely deironed! Now I go four times a year, and keep a check on iron levels.

Here's the best part: my periods have returned. I'm back exercising again, working full time. . . . Even my arthritis has improved. My sister Joyce is still struggling with diabetes, and the iron damage to her pancreas seems permanent. I was very lucky that Joyce was diagnosed. We both were lucky. I know that most people never receive a correct diagnosis.

I'm glad I made up my mind to put up with intensive treatment. The reward of enjoying a healthy existence is the best reward of all!

If you have hemochromatosis or if someone close to you has it, please know that it CAN get better. I know. I've lived it first hand.

The Iron Overload Diseases Association is hoping that the awareness of hemochromatosis in women will be improved. Since hemochromatosis is a genetic disease, the bad gene is distributed equally among men and women. Hemochromatosis does seem to strike men more severely, though experts are not sure why. But the male/female ratio of diagnosed hemochromatosis victims is nowhere near the ten-to-one estimate printed in many medical texts: the association estimates that it is more like 1.4 to 1.

Subtle Signs

As you could see from the two examples above, amenorrhea is often an early sign of hemochromatosis in women. Likewise, impotence is often observed in men before more severe symptoms appear. There is an interesting case of a thirty-year-old man whose sexual function was completely normal for most of his life. He had fathered a child when he was twenty-six and had enjoyed excellent health. He then noticed diminished sexual desire, followed by reduced volume of ejaculate and then impotence. When he was referred to a major teaching hospital, his case was used as an example for medical students and published in an influential journal.[12] A notable feature of this case is that the initial diagnosis was completely wrong.

On examination, the doctors noticed that the man was losing body hair, his testes were small, and his male hormone levels were low. His liver function tests were abnormal. The man also complained that his strength had diminished and he had recently developed arthritis in one shoulder as well as in his hands, feet, knees, and ankles.

An expert endocrinologist filled several pages with his account of what could be wrong with the man. Buried in the middle of this long essay is a brief note that hemochromatosis could damage the pituitary and lead to these symptoms. The endocrinologist deserves credit for this and for one other thing: he noted that he would need blood-iron measurements to exclude hemochromatosis confidently. But he thought that the absence of bronze skin or diabetic symptoms, classical signs of hemochromatosis, went against this diagnosis, so he went on to look for other causes. His final diagnosis, some obscure form of inherited liver disease, was wrong: the patient had hemochromatosis, as was proven later by serum iron measurements and a liver biopsy.

This case shows how doctors still use some of the classic signs of hemochromatosis to rule out the disease. But more often than not, more subtle signs, such as impotence and arthritis, are most important. In addition to the fact that all of us need to check our iron levels periodically, anyone with arthritis, impotence, amenorrhea, or liver abnormalities clearly needs to check them as well.[11]

Medical Malpractice

The mishandling of hemochromatosis patients has led to several lawsuits in the past five years. The first, settled in 1985, was John Mury's, as related at the beginning of this chapter. Five other cases have been settled, all in favor of the hemochromatosis victims, and twelve are now believed to be pending. In every case, the charges against the doctors centered on the failure to diagnose the disease. In every case, the patients hoped the word would get out that doctors should pay more attention to iron levels and the potential for hemochromatosis.[6]

The latest case to be settled was for the largest sum yet: over one million dollars. This case involved a manager at a large company who suffered from liver disease for many years. His doctors failed to bring the results of his abnormal liver tests to his attention, and his condition, compounded by incapacitating arthritis, deteriorated to the point that he had to quit work. When he finally found out that hemochromatosis was the cause of his abnormal test results, he couldn't believe it. He told me bitterly, "My kids could have read that liver test." He also mentioned that he thinks that patients should always get copies of test results and question their doctors on the possible causes of any abnormal readings.

The Awareness Gap

These stories show that hemochromatosis victims often fall between the cracks in our health care system. What has gone wrong? Why is it so difficult for the medical community to diagnose a fairly straightforward disease?

Surely the iron-is-only-good-for-you myth must have contributed to this state of affairs. We have seen how freely some doctors prescribe iron for various complaints, even without testing iron levels beforehand. The old Geritol commercials, the iron-equals-strength notion, and other cultural influences have had their effect on doctors as well as patients.

Another reason why hemochromatosis often goes undetected

is that doctors can assume that the liver damage seen in this disease is due to excessive alcohol ingestion. As you have heard in the preceding stories, doctors often question the patients closely about their drinking habits, and sometimes they are satisfied with the more common diagnosis of alcohol-induced cirrhosis instead of searching for other causes. Several hemochromatosis patients I talked to were frustrated when their doctors failed to believe that they were light drinkers.

In addition to roadblocks in our health care system, there is an extremely low degree of awareness about hemochromatosis for a disease so common. Part of this has to do with the fact that we have only known how prevalent the disease is for a few years. It may take a new generation of doctors, armed with more accurate pictures of both iron and hemochromatosis, to improve the situation.

Hemochromatosis victims also say that the disease has a certain stigma attached to it, and perhaps this might prevent people from speaking out and spreading the word. Some iron-overload patients feel that the bad gene has "marked" them for life, and they do not want it publicized. Those who suffer from impotence or amenorrhea worry that their privacy might be compromised. Perhaps for these reasons, the handful of celebrities and public figures who are known to have hemochromatosis have not yet given one of their most valuable gifts to society: their unique ability to draw attention to a worthy cause.

Hope for the Future

The Iron Overload Diseases Association and a second organization, the Hemochromatosis Research Foundation, based in Albany, New York, continue to work diligently to increase the awareness of the public and the medical community. (The founder and president of the latter organization is Dr. Margaret A. Krikker, the physician who led the fight against excessive iron fortification of flour.) Though always running on tight budgets, these organizations, together with their medical and scientific advisors, have done a remarkable job in providing information to patients and families and in organizing international conferences to stimulate research and to educate doctors. In addition, the week of September 11–17 each year has been designated as Iron Overload Diseases Week.[6] And, as noted at the end of the previous chapter, some progress is being made toward getting warning labels on high-iron products. These labels may save lives not only by protecting those with hemochromatosis but also by publicizing the disease itself and encouraging more people to ask their doctors about it.

At the time of this writing, another promising step has been taken in the right direction. Metpath, Inc., one of the major blood-screening companies, has added an effective set of iron tests to its routine Chem-Screen laboratory analysis. Preliminary results indicate that roughly 1 percent of the population, potentially 2.4 million Americans, have elevated iron levels. If other companies follow this action, thousands of hemochromatosis victims will be diagnosed early, and for many of them, significant organ damage may be prevented.

The greatest hope, however, is that medical research will progress to the point where we will be able to correct inherited diseases directly by altering a person's recipe cards or genes in certain cells of the body. This twenty-first-century technology is still many years away, but it is an exciting hope for the future. In the shorter term, perhaps three to five years, this research may provide important tests to identify hemochromatosis directly by locating the damaged gene in unknowing victims. If these people can be diagnosed early, before the presentation of any symptoms, they are likely to lead long, rust-free lives.

8

Other Causes of Iron Overload

In addition to hereditary hemochromatosis, there are other ways in which people can become overloaded with iron. In this chapter, we'll look at three examples where excess iron is obtained from cooking food in iron pots, chronic ingestion of iron supplements, or multiple blood transfusions. While these cases deal with only certain groups of people, they nevertheless offer important lessons for all of us. The first two cases, dealing with excessive ingestion of iron, are particularly important because they show that "normal" folks, people without inherited defects in iron metabolism, are not protected from iron overload.

Iron and the South African Bantus

During the years 1924–1928, A. S. Strachan of Glasgow, Scotland, was researching the health of blacks in Johannesburg, South Africa.[1,2] In collecting information for his medical thesis, he found that a large proportion of blacks in the hospitals had severe degrees of iron overload. He later reported that roughly half of 745 autopsies performed on deceased black patients showed excess iron in the liver, spleen, and other organs. Ten percent had liver cirrhosis and 3 percent had liver cancer. For unknown reasons, iron, either directly or indirectly, seemed to be an important cause of death for blacks, especially those that spoke the language known as Bantu.

The Bantu-speaking people represent the majority of blacks in South Africa. They are thought to be descendants of a proud and powerful tribe that migrated into southern Africa and spread its culture and language throughout the region. Was there something peculiar in their customs that led to iron overload?

The Bantu diet did not seem out of the ordinary. Eating did have a special meaning to the Bantus: in the Bantu language, the verb *to live* is the same as the verb *to eat*. And they were especially fond of meat, a good source of iron, when they could get it. They even had a special word, *kashia*, for "meat hunger," and they had a tendency to go on "meat orgies" after a good hunt.[3,4] But simple measurements of the iron content in their diet, which largely consisted of grains, indicated that their overall iron intake from foods was quite typical of other cultures.

The breakthrough in understanding the cause of the Bantu form of iron overload came when in 1950 some scientists measured iron content *after* the foods were cooked. The Bantus, as do many other primitive cultures, use iron pots for almost all their cooking, and large quantities of iron leach out and dissolve in their foods. By itself, the food would have provided the Bantu roughly 10–30 milligrams of iron per day; after cooking, however, their daily intake rose to 100–200 milligrams. This is equivalent to taking large doses of iron supplements every day for life.

Home-Brewed Beer

While the iron content of cooked food certainly contributed to iron overload in the Bantus, scientists found that their home-brewed beer, also prepared in iron pots, was the worst offender.[1,2] The Bantu were adept at preparing fermented beverages; they made ten types of beer. They often had miniature "breweries" right outside their grass and mud huts. They were not teetotalers. An anthropologist once wrote, "It is no meaningless alliteration to speak of 'the Boozy Bantu' whose love of beer can only be compared with the Scotchman's reputed love of whisky and the Dutchman's penchant for gin."[3]

Bantu beer is a high-iron tonic. First, the beer itself is acidic, and this helps dissolve the iron from the pots in which it is prepared. Second, the alcohol enhances iron absorption in the gut. And finally, the substances present in grains that normally inhibit iron absorption are to some degree removed in the brewing process.

Analysis of Bantu beers showed an average iron concentration of about 40 milligrams per liter. Since the alcohol content is low, many Bantus would drink two or more liters per day, leading to daily iron intakes of 80 milligrams or more.

For years the Bantus have been poisoning themselves with iron in this fashion. Their ancestors were known for their skill in metallurgy, particularly in ironworking. In an odd way, this skill has had dire consequences for the health of this important and populous tribe.

Scientists believe that over the years the situation has improved for many of the Bantus. Modern pots and conventionally prepared beverages have replaced the crude pots and dangerous traditional brews. As a result, the incidence of iron overload in Johannesburg is thought to have decreased by 50 percent over the last twenty-five to thirty years.[2]

The example of Bantu iron overload is an important one. It shows the effect of cooking in iron pots—throw yours away! It also shows that the chronic ingestion of excess iron, even in the absence of hereditary disorders like hemochromatosis, can lead to liver damage, diabetes and even death.

Self- or Doctor-Induced Iron Overload

Those pretty pink iron pills so often prescribed for "anemic" women are not innocent. These supplements contain large amounts of iron—100 milligrams or more—similar to the quantities ingested daily by the Bantus. While these pills should be reserved for special cases of severe iron deficiency or for use during pregnancy, people often continue to take them for many years, either voluntarily or on the advice of a physician.

From several reports in the medical literature, a composite picture of self-induced iron poisoning materializes.[5-8] It is usually discovered in a middle-aged or elderly woman who began to take iron quite early in life for anemia. Unfortunately, a serum iron test is never performed to see if the patient really needs iron at all.

The reports tell us that the woman continues taking iron pills for ten, twenty, even fifty years. She then seeks professional help for either fatigue or progressive ill health. Sometimes she or her family have noted the characteristic brown spots or tanning that is often present in hereditary hemochromatosis.

The doctor invariably finds an enlarged liver, signifying liver damage from the excess iron. Evidence of diabetes or other abnormalities may also be present. On careful examination, the doctor will also find the very high serum iron values characteristic of iron overload.

In those cases where the doctor is enlightened, the patient is treated as if she had hereditary hemochromatosis. The excess iron is removed by phlebotomy. However, in most cases, the liver disease progresses unabated, and the patient may die of cirrhosis or heart disease.

What about short-term iron supplementation? Many of us have taken iron supplements for a period of time and appear to suffer no adverse effects. Surely it is the long-term iron accumulation that affected the women described above. However, a 1984 West German study showed that short-term supplementation (twelve weeks) with the most common form of iron pills can lead to mild liver damage.[9-11] While this was a small study and needs to be confirmed on a larger scale, clearly there is more than enough evidence that people do not need excess iron.

Acute iron poisoning should also be mentioned. There are about two thousand cases each year, primarily in young children who are attracted to the candylike appearance of the iron supplement pills. As few as two tablets can cause severe poisoning, and three to six can cause death. Within thirty minutes to an hour after ingestion, children experience abdominal pain and may vomit the stomach contents, which appear brown or reddish-brown. Hyperventilation and heart trouble can begin soon thereafter, and without treatment, death may come within four to six hours.

Iron Death From Blood Transfusions

The damaging effects of excess iron are also seen in patients who must receive repeated blood transfusions. Since each unit of blood contains more than 200 milligrams of red-cell iron, and since the body lacks an efficient iron excretion mechanism, iron overload develops quite rapidly in these patients.

The most common diseases which require frequent transfusions are those in which hemoglobin, the oxygen-carrying pigment in the blood, is not synthesized or is defective. The most important of these is *beta-thalassemia*, also known as Cooley's anemia, an inherited disease that is prevalent in people of Mediterranean or Southeast Asian descent. Roughly one in four hundred people in these groups can acquire this tragic disease. The inheritance pattern is identical to that of hereditary hemochromatosis. If both parents silently carry the abnormal gene for beta-thalassemia, there is a 25 percent chance that each child will inherit two copies of the defective gene.

The iron buildup in beta-thalassemia is quite severe. In addition to the iron in the transfused blood, the bone marrow cells, which are futilely trying to make hemoglobin, signal that more iron is needed, resulting in the increased absorption of iron from the diet.

In beta-thalassemia, patients suffer many of the consequences experienced by people with the full-blown form of hereditary hemochromatosis, including liver and heart failure and diabetes. They often die in their teens or early twenties.

There is hope for advancements in the treatment of beta-thalassemia and similar diseases. In the future, we may be able to replace the defective gene and completely cure these victims. For now, these patients have to be repeatedly injected with substances which remove the excess iron. The search is on for orally active drugs with fewer side effects.

Something Old, Something New

In hospital beds in small Mediterranean or African villages or even in your local community, iron is taking its toll. Massive amounts of iron, either from inherited disorders or self-induced, rust the human body from the inside out. These are medical facts written on thousands of pages of respected medical journals: that, in massive quantities, iron kills is something we have known for years.

In the next part of this book, a new slant on the iron story will be discussed: even moderately elevated levels of iron, far less than that in true iron overload, may be endangering your health.

Part 4

EVEN MODERATELY ELEVATED IRON LEVELS MAY BE DANGEROUS TO YOUR HEALTH

9

Iron and Heart Disease

By now you are a virtual expert on iron metabolism and iron-overload disease. Having read the first eight chapters of this book, you may know more about iron than some doctors. Examples of iron overload, especially hereditary hemochromatosis, are important to understand on your way to becoming iron-balanced. Obviously, if you have signs of hemochromatosis, you should be screened for this disease as soon as possible. But the odds are that you are free of this or any of the other forms of overt iron overload, and therefore we should turn our attention to the potential dangers of even moderately elevated iron levels.

The Iron-Depletion Hypothesis

Here in Part 4 are discussed the growing links between moderate levels of iron and aging, as well as moderate levels of iron and the diseases that concern you and your family the most—heart disease, brain disorders, and cancer. At the end of this part of the book, I describe a relatively new medical hypothesis—the iron-depletion hypothesis—that ties all this information together. This theory states that all of us, men and women, would be healthiest if we maintain fairly low iron levels, perhaps as low as that of most women prior to menopause. This is quite easy to do using the guidelines in Part 5.

The idea that we would be better off maintaining lower iron levels is not entirely new, though it is doubtful that your doctor will know much about it. Like any medical hypothesis, this one will have its ups and downs through the years as scientists refine their ideas. Two things are clear for now: first, the dangerous role that iron often plays in our tissues is becoming increasingly apparent, both in animal and in human studies; second, the iron-depletion hypothesis makes good sense.

The commonsense approach to proper iron balance is identical to our modern approach towards cholesterol. As the links between cholesterol and cardiovascular disease became clear throughout the twentieth century, it was obvious that very high levels of cholesterol, such as those exhibited by people with certain inherited diseases, are extremely dangerous. It was also found that even moderately high levels of cholesterol can lead to higher rates of heart disease. Likewise, the high iron levels found in hereditary hemochromatosis clearly cause death and disability. Why wouldn't moderately high levels of iron be dangerous as well?

Heart Disease: Risk Factors and Unanswered Questions

Heart disease is the major killer in the U.S. and the world as a whole. The dominant form of heart disease that all of us worry about is coronary artery disease. In this condition, the inside diameter of the coronary arteries—which literally carry the life-blood of the heart—become narrowed, reducing blood flow and the supply of oxygen to the heart muscle. If a small blood clot happens to lodge in the narrowed opening, the entire blood supply to one or more regions of the heart is cut off, and a heart attack results.

As you are well aware, doctors have figured out that there are a number of controllable risk factors for this disease, and we are constantly reminded that we should be keeping an eye on these. They include cholesterol, the favorite of many doctors and certain "health-minded" food companies, as well as blood pressure, obesity, smoking, and exercise. In short, we are better off with less of the first four and more of the fifth.

Now, if we took a group of people, analyzed their risk factors, and followed their incidence of heart disease, we ought to be able to construct a strong, mathematical relationship: those with better scores on their risk-factor charts should have a lower incidence of heart disease. As it turns out, this works to some degree, but many doctors and scientists have been disappointed with the results of these studies. While the studies certainly give us an idea of what we should be controlling to minimize the risk of heart disease, there are so many cases in which the analysis does not work that many scientists believe we are missing the full picture. These investigators continue to look for other risk factors. Iron may be a missing piece of this puzzle.

In the following pages you will learn how an analysis of iron levels may help to explain some of the most perplexing questions related to heart disease today. These questions include:

- Why do men have more heart attacks than women?
- Why do heart disease rates rapidly increase in women after menopause?
- Why do aspirin, fish oil, vegetarian diets, and exercise protect the heart?

The Bell Tolls for Men

The first question relating to the higher rate of heart disease in men is of fundamental importance both in understanding the nature of the disease and in figuring out why the members of the female sex enjoy the special gift of longevity. Heart disease is the major contributor to the "gender gap" in life expectancy. The World Health Organization estimates that the life expectancy for women born in the U.S. in 1986 is 78.6 years, some seven years longer than men (71.4 years). It is largely heart disease that robs the "average man" of those seven precious years.[1]

The relatively early death of men in our society has important social and economic costs.[2,3] Current projections for the U.S. reveal that in 2010, in the eighty-five-and-older age bracket there will be 266 women for every 100 men. Just think of the increased enjoyment and quality of life an elderly woman would experience if the heart disease rates in men could be reduced to that of women, resulting in more comparable life expectancies. This may also reduce certain economic hardships, since couples can often provide for themselves better than either partner could alone.

Why Is the Female Heart Spared?

When it comes to heart disease, men need to become more like women, particularly younger women. Women experience a far lower rate of heart disease than men, until they reach menopause, at which time their heart disease rate begins to approach that of men.[4] This magical protection offered to the female sex has puzzled doctors for years. They have come up with many explanations, but none of these theories seem to stand the test of time.

The most popular notion is that women possess some sort of hormonal protection. Hormones are substances that communicate important messages between different organs, messages dealing with sexual characteristics, cell growth, and other processes. Women possess a different set of hormones than men, and this may be an important factor in determining their relative susceptibility to many diseases. But the possible link between female hormones and heart disease is currently a muddled picture.

Most of the attention has focused on the female hormone called estrogen. When women reach menopause, their ovaries secrete lower amounts of estrogen. This is often thought to be linked with the higher incidence of heart disease in older women. According to this notion, the total absence of estrogen in men would lead to their high rate of heart disease at all ages.

Since many women take estrogen in their postmenopausal years, it has become possible to study the effects of estrogen replacement therapy on the incidence of heart disease. Indeed, some studies have shown that estrogen is beneficial for women. However, what is good for the goose is not good for the gander. In an early effort to "make men more like women," the female hormone was administered to men with alarming results: it *increased* the heart attack rate![5]

An Early Clue

A further indication that something was wrong with the estrogen theory came in the famous Framingham Heart Study, which followed heart disease incidence in four thousand residents of Framingham, Massachusetts.[6] In agreement with other studies, the investigators found an increased risk of heart disease in women within two years after menopause. The key result, however, involved the comparison of heart disease rates in two subgroups of women: those that had hysterectomies (removal of the uterus, or womb) without the removal of the estrogen-producing ovaries, and those that had both operations simultaneously. On the basis of the estrogen protection theory, you would expect the latter group to have higher heart attack rates. However, *both* groups had a similar increase in risk compared to premenopausal women. Somehow the removal of the uterus, not the ovaries, strips women of their natural protection.[7]

The Framingham researchers concluded:[6]

> We can only speculate as to the reasons for the postmenopausal increase in coronary heart disease incidence. Natural hormonal changes occurring with menopause are exceedingly complex; we cannot clearly specify which, if any, lead to a rise in coronary heart disease incidence. . . . A careful investigation of this subject may lead to a better

understanding of the factors that account for the remarkable protection against coronary heart disease enjoyed by premenopausal women. Somewhere in this tantalizing mystery may lie a lesson of profound importance in understanding the genesis and course of this disease, perhaps in men as well as women.

Iron: The Missing Link

A resolution of this important question in heart disease has been offered by Dr. Jerome Sullivan, a professor of pathology at the Medical University of South Carolina and a leader in the area of iron–heart disease links. Free of the conventional patterns of thought in cardiology, Dr. Sullivan looked for nonhormonal explanations for the Framingham results. He directly addressed the following questions: Why was the removal of the uterus, or its dysfunction at menopause, important in increasing heart disease risk? Is it menstruation and the blood loss thereof that protects women from heart attacks?

It was Dr. Sullivan who first proposed that the protection exhibited by premenopausal women might be due to their lower bodily iron loads, which result from regular blood loss. He noted that the different patterns of iron accumulation in men and women seemed to mirror trends in heart-disease mortality rates.[7]

Take a look at Figure 9-1, a simple version of data presented by Dr. Sullivan in a 1989 issue of the *American Heart Journal*. Here we are plotting, as a function of age, the values of storage iron, heart-disease mortality rates, and total cholesterol levels in terms of male-to-female ratios of these values. The plot for iron levels shows that men twenty to forty years old have three to four times the amount of stored iron as women; as women reach menopause (age forty-five to fifty) and begin to accumulate iron, the male-to-female ratio drops to one or two.

Now look at the strikingly similar plot for heart-disease mortality rates. Men thirty to fifty years old have roughly four times the mortality rate of women, in close agreement with the ratio

Figure 9-1. Heart disease rates and iron and cholesterol levels in men and women as a function of age. The top two graphs show that the difference between the iron levels of men and women as they age has a similar pattern to the difference in heart-disease mortality rates. The quantities shown are ratios calculated by taking, for each age group, the iron level, heart disease rate, and cholesterol level for males and dividing by the corresponding value for females. Men aged twenty-five to forty-five accumulate iron more rapidly than women in the same age group, most of whom are menstruating, resulting in high male/female iron-level ratios of 3–4. This is comparable to the heart disease ratios of 4–4.5. When women reach menopause, they begin to accumulate iron rapidly, and thus the male/female iron-level ratio decreases from age forty-five; a similar decrease in the heart disease ratio is present. The bottom graph shows that variations in cholesterol levels are unlikely to be the basis of the male-female difference in heart disease rates. (Adapted from Sullivan, J. L. "The Iron Paradigm of Ischemic Heart Disease." *American Heart Journal* 117 [1989]: 1177–1188.)

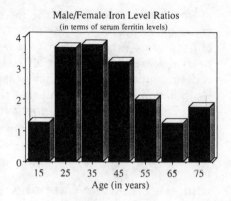

Male/Female Iron Level Ratios
(in terms of serum ferritin levels)

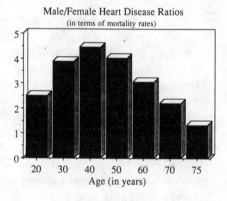

Male/Female Heart Disease Ratios
(in terms of mortality rates)

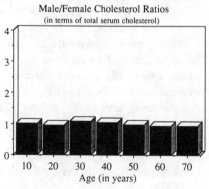

Male/Female Cholesterol Ratios
(in terms of total serum cholesterol)

of iron levels. In addition, the male-female mortality ratio decreases with age, just as the plot of iron ratios does.

These data establish iron as a new potential risk factor for heart disease. The data are of course indirect and will need further confirmation, but they make good sense. In addition, Dr. Sullivan has pointed out that the proposed role of iron in heart disease helps explain other perplexing observations. Let's look at a couple of these.

Cholesterol Alone Cannot Kill

Look back at the plot at the bottom of Figure 9-1. This shows the ratio of male cholesterol levels to female levels. The data are plotted on the same scale as the preceding data on heart disease deaths and iron to emphasize the tiny and most likely insignificant differences in cholesterol levels that exist. If one examines the average levels of other cholesterol indices—low-density lipoprotein, or "bad" cholesterol, and high-density lipoprotein, "good" cholesterol—and various ratios thereof, similar plots are obtained. Though cholesterol is undoubtedly involved in blocking the coronary arteries, the relative levels of this substance in the blood cannot account for the large differences in heart disease between men and women.

A second piece of evidence to consider involves heart disease in women with *familial hypercholesterolemia*, or FH, an inherited disease marked by elevated levels of serum cholesterol. The full-blown form of this disease occurs when both sets of genes inherited from the parents contain the genetic defect (the homozygous state). Cholesterol levels are some six to eight times the normal level, and even young children often suffer heart attacks. In the mild form of FH, where only one set of bad genes is inherited (the heterozygous state), cholesterol levels are two to three times normal; these individuals provide a more useful and realistic model of the effects of elevated cholesterol.

The occurrence of heart disease in individuals with heterozygous FH follows a pattern that is similar to that of the general population. While FH men have higher incidence of disease than normal men, FH women are apparently protected until meno-pause, when the incidence increases.[7] Is it not strange in our "cholesterol age" that these FH women have high cholesterol levels—but the same incidence of heart disease as unaffected women? I think we have to move into a new Iron Age to explain this phenomenon.

Lessons From the Seventh-Day Adventists

An additional piece of evidence against cholesterol as an all-important cause of heart disease comes from the studies of Seventh-Day Adventist men in the U.S., Norway, and the Netherlands. The members of this religious denomination, three million worldwide, follow church proscriptions regarding ab-stention from smoking and drinking alcoholic beverages. They also may follow the church's recommendation of a lacto-ovo vegetarian diet. This type of diet excludes meat, fish, and poultry but does include some high-cholesterol foods such as dairy prod-ucts and eggs.

Researchers have wondered for some time why Adventist men exhibit 40–50 percent fewer heart disease–related deaths than non-Adventist men, far lower than would be expected on the basis of their nonsmoking status alone. It has long been known that vegetarians exhibit reduced heart-disease mortality rates, and this has usually been ascribed to reductions in cholesterol levels. However, the Adventist men, even though they abstain from eating meat, still get a lot of cholesterol and saturated fat from their high intake of dairy products. Indeed, studies have shown that their blood-cholesterol levels are only slightly lower than those of other men, roughly 6 percent, far too small a difference to account for the dramatically lower heart disease rates.[8]

A more likely explanation for the protection exhibited by Ad-ventist men is that their lower intake of high-iron meat leads to lower body-iron stores.[9] While studies of the iron levels in these men have not yet been reported, it is a fairly safe guess that their iron levels are lower than those of carnivorous men. Several studies of vegetarians, including studies of other groups of lacto-ovo vegetarians, have shown significant drops in iron levels.

Cholesterol *and* Iron: The Combined Risk Factor

In heart disease, it appears that there are essentially two dominant, diet-related risk factors: cholesterol *and* iron. The Adventist men may have reduced the risk of heart attack by modifying one of these, their iron levels, by eating a vegetarian diet. One wonders how low the risk would be if they cut down on eggs and high-fat dairy products, thereby lowering their cholesterol levels as well.

We can get an idea of how effective the lowering of *both* cholesterol and iron levels might be by examining heart-disease mortality rates in different countries. Though such comparisons can never stand as absolute epidemiologic proof due to the problem in comparing people from different racial and social backgrounds, they have provided grounds for many of the concepts in heart disease prevention, particularly the importance of low cholesterol levels. The question for now is, do populations in countries with low-fat *and* low-iron diets exhibit lower heart disease rates?

In 1989 I collected available data on the average cholesterol and iron levels in men and women in different countries and compared these data with reported coronary-artery-disease mortality rates. The results of this analysis, published in 1991 in the international journal *Medical Hypotheses*, showed that heart-disease mortality rates correlated better with a combination of iron and cholesterol values than with either index alone.[10] Let's take a look at some of the data.

For simplicity, let's focus on Japanese, Venezuelan, and U.S. men. As you can see in Figure 9-2, a plot of their coronary-artery-disease mortality rates looks like a staircase: the Japanese men have the lowest level of heart disease, the U.S. men the most, and the Venezuelan men are in between. Right below this plot of mortality rates is a similar plot of cholesterol levels in these men. There certainly is no agreement between these first two plots. The latter shows the Venezuelan men to have the lowest cholesterol levels, yet they have much higher heart disease rates than Japanese men.

A plot of the iron levels in these men shows a somewhat better relationship to the mortality data than the cholesterol plot, with the Japanese men exhibiting the lowest iron levels and the lowest heart disease rate. However, there is some disagreement in the Venezuelan-U.S. comparison: the values used for iron levels in this analysis (liver iron content) were higher for Venezuelan men, but their mortality rate is less than U.S. men.

But, if we look at a combination of iron and cholesterol values by multiplying the two numbers, a much better relationship is obtained. The bottom right plot in Figure 9-2 shows the staircase increase noted in the plot of the mortality rates. In this example, and in the full analysis recently published, it appears that the highest mortality rate occurs in men like those in the U.S. (as well as England, Australia, and many northern European countries) where *both* iron and cholesterol levels are relatively high. A moderate level of heart disease mortality is seen in South or Central American groups like the Venezuelans. While these groups exhibit very low cholesterol levels, even lower than the Japanese, their heart disease rates are still moderately high, perhaps due to their relatively high iron levels. (One wonders whether the consumption of relatively high-iron red wine in these cultures might contribute to their high iron levels.)

Clearly the best of both worlds is exhibited by the Japanese men who have long been examined for the reasons underlying their low rate of heart disease. The Japanese seem to represent the ideal state of relatively low cholesterol *and* low iron levels, presumably stemming from their relatively healthy diet that has little red meat or dairy products and plenty of fish and vegetables.

You can see that the inclusion of iron as a potential risk factor for heart disease helps us explain a number of observations that have puzzled investigators for years. Cholesterol levels are only part of the puzzle, and iron may be one of the most important missing pieces. The low iron levels in premenopausal women, the Japanese, and perhaps the Adventist men seem to protect

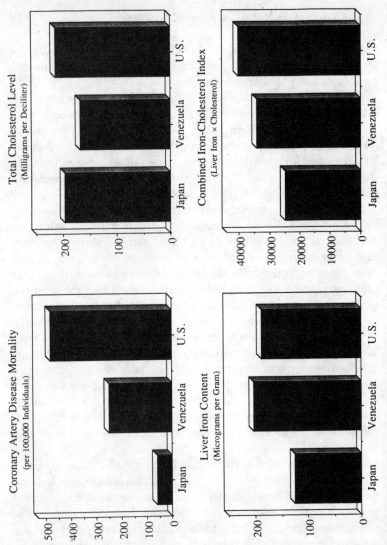

Figure 9-2. Heart disease rates and iron and cholesterol levels in three countries. These graphs compare the coronary-artery-disease rates in men from three countries to corresponding cholesterol, iron, and iron-cholesterol levels. While variations in cholesterol levels and liver iron levels (a good estimate of iron stores) do not individually correspond to the proportionally lower rates of coronary artery disease in Japan and Venezuela, the combined index, liver iron multiplied by cholesterol, does.

them from this disease, independent of their respective cholesterol levels.

Iron Cannonballs and Damage to the Heart Muscle

Now if these studies based on populations were all we had to go on, the iron–heart disease link would be provocative but perhaps not that persuasive. However, further support for this theory has come from more direct, biochemical investigations performed in recent years.

The most important group of these studies, performed at Johns Hopkins and several other universities, has shown that iron is involved in damaging the heart muscle when the blood supply is temporarily cut off and then resumed.[7,11,12] Blockage in a coronary artery can occur in a full-fledged heart attack or in transient "mini-attacks" which may or may not present physical symptoms such as angina. Paradoxically, the heart suffers little when the supply of oxygen is diminished; the real damage is done when fresh oxygen once again flows through the arteries.

The damage to the heart muscle appears to involve that dangerous combination of iron and oxygen that was discussed in Chapter 2. When blood flow is cut off, the biochemical condition within the heart cells is altered. This causes iron to be released from the large "storage bin" molecules of ferritin like cannonballs from an arsenal. It is a potentially explosive situation, biochemically speaking. When blood flow is resumed and oxygen reenters the cells, a wild, uncontrolled degradation process known as *iron-catalyzed oxidation* is unleashed, and the muscle fibers and cell walls suffer severe, often irreparable damage.

Much of the evidence supporting this sequence of events comes from animal studies of the effects of different drugs on tissue damage from induced heart attacks. The role of iron has been most clearly demonstrated when a special iron-sequestering drug known as *desferrioxamine* is administered in these experiments. This drug essentially wraps around each of the iron cannonballs and prevents them from initiating the degradation process. Several different investigations have shown that this drug reduces the tissue damage considerably.

While studies with this iron-sequestering drug have not yet been performed in humans, there is a very recent human study showing that the tissue-oxidation process does occur when blood flow is restored to the oxygen-starved heart. Performed by a group of investigators in London and published in the British journal *Lancet*, this study found chemical evidence that this process occurred in the blood of patients after their clogged arteries were opened with a clot-busting drug called *streptokinase*.[13] Further studies should clarify the role of iron in this process.

Iron and Your Pipes

A second possible role for iron in heart disease is in assisting the artery-clogging process. We tend to see this process as a plumbing problem, like a clogged drain, resulting from a high level of cholesterol in the blood, which accumulates on the artery wall. However, this disease, called *atherosclerosis*, is much more complicated than that. As we learn more about it, we can see how iron may be involved.

Atherosclerosis is not so much a clogging process as it is a disease of the pipes—the arteries—themselves. A certain form of cholesterol known as low-density lipoprotein or LDL, the "bad" form of cholesterol, gets trapped by cells in the artery wall. These and other cells in the wall gradually enlarge or multiply to the point that they begin to decrease the size of the interior of the artery. This leads to diminished blood supply to the heart and the potential for a heart attack.

Recent studies suggest that the key step in this process is the trapping of LDL by cells in the artery wall. Dr. Daniel Steinberg and Dr. Sampath Parthasarathy and their colleagues at the University of California at San Diego have shown that the "bad" cholesterol must be oxidized before the artery cells will trap it. The type of cells that perform this are in a way like little garbage cans, picking up the rancid cholesterol.[14]

Iron is most likely involved in this oxidation of "bad" cholesterol. In fact, researchers in the field cannot even get cholesterol oxidized efficiently in the test tube without adding tiny quantities of iron or other metallic substances that assist in the degradation process. In addition, recent evidence indicates that iron assists the bad cholesterol in actually killing artery cells.[15] Though the details of this process are still being worked out, the fact that iron plays a significant role in coronary narrowing—the very beginning of most forms of heart disease—is likely to emerge.

New Explanations for Old Remedies and Curses

It appears that iron has you coming and going. With roles in the artery-narrowing process and the muscle damage that eventually results, iron appears to be involved at both the beginning and the end of heart disease. Clearly, any life-style or dietary factors that raise your iron level may increase your risk of heart attack. Conversely, a reduction in bodily iron load for those that have high levels may decrease risk. Let's look at a number of these factors in the light of the new iron–heart disease link. As was first recognized by Dr. Jerome Sullivan, alterations in iron levels can explain many of the effects of these factors on heart disease rates.[7]

Oral Contraceptives. Numerous studies have shown that prolonged use of oral contraceptives, which contain synthetic sex hormones, significantly increases a woman's chance of having a heart attack. The increased risk extends even into the menopause years, when oral contraceptives are no longer taken. Until recently, no comprehensive explanation for this serious side effect has been offered.

The iron-heart link provides us with the answer. As described further in Chapter 15, it is well known that oral contraceptives decrease menstrual blood flow in most women to a third or half the normal rate. Women who use oral contraceptives are more likely to build up their iron stores earlier in life. This has been confirmed in recent studies, which show that the amount of storage iron in women who had been using oral contraceptives for two years or more is roughly double that of nonusers. Thus, oral contraceptives partially rob younger women of the peculiar protection—the effect of iron loss through menstruation—with which they are uniquely blessed. The higher iron levels in these women may be what increases their risk of heart attack.

Inherited Factors. Heart disease, in particular an early onset form that preferentially attacks many men under the age of fifty, tends to run in families. While there are several inherited disorders dealing with cholesterol metabolism, the prevalence of these conditions is far too low to account for the rate of family-related heart attacks in middle-aged men. Investigators continue to look for the unknown genetic factors at work.

Dr. Sullivan has proposed that the mild form of hereditary hemochromatosis, the iron-overload disease, may be one such inherited factor that predisposes a significant fraction of our population to premature heart attacks. As you recall from Chapter 7, this form of hemochromatosis is characterized by moderate increases in storage iron, particularly in men. As we begin to learn more, we may be able to screen people for this disease and look directly at whether those that carry this trait are at higher risk, as we expect.

An Aspirin a Day. Those common white pills, the most heavily used pharmaceutical in the world, have been shown in some studies to be effective in preventing heart attacks. While there is still controversy as to aspirin's effectiveness and who should be taking it, most cardiologists are firm believers in this drug: it has been estimated that over 40 percent of them take it at least every other day.[16]

Aspirin is thought to "thin the blood" by reducing the formation of blood clots that trigger heart attacks. However, aspirin's effectiveness could also be due to reductions in iron loads. You see, aspirin irritates the stomachs of many people, and whether they know it or not, they lose significant amounts of blood through the stomach (and into the bowel) with each aspirin tablet. With an aspirin a day, the blood—and iron—losses could equal those of menstruation. Taking aspirin could essentially convert the iron metabolism of a man or postmenopausal woman to that of a younger, menstruating woman in whom heart attacks are extremely rare.

A Fish a Day. The Greenland Eskimos provided the modern medical world with one of the more intriguing concepts in heart disease prevention. Investigators found that their regular consumption of deepwater fish seemed to be linked to their low rate of heart disease.

The key component in deepwater fish is thought to be a special fatty substance, an omega-3 fatty acid known as *eicosapentaenoic acid,* or EPA, which you can now get in capsule form from your local health food store. Like aspirin, this substance reduces the clotting ability of the blood, and it is this that most scientists think is responsible for the protection provided to the heart. If this were the sole explanation, you might expect that even short-term use of fish oil would be effective in preventing heart disease. However, investigators have found no evidence for important short-term benefits, and it appears that the oil must be consumed regularly for years or even decades before the benefits are apparent.

These observations are consistent with the idea that, as with aspirin, the preventative effects of fish oil stem from chronic blood and iron loss. If the blood is "thinned out," tiny spots of bleeding in the stomach and intestines (which occur naturally quite often) will not heal as quickly, and more blood will be lost than normal. Over years, this would be expected to reduce iron loads, leading to possible health benefits exhibited by Eskimos and other fish-eating peoples. A study of iron metabolism in these people is needed to resolve this issue.

Exercise. A final heart disease prevention technique which may work in part by lowering iron levels is exercise. Exercise has long been known to be good for the heart, though doctors cannot seem to agree on why this should be so. I became interested in whether the beneficial effects of exercise might be due in part to changes in iron levels. As I explain further in Chapter 19, there is considerable evidence that this indeed may be the case. Briefly, exercise leads to a reduction in your iron levels via blood loss in the gastrointestinal tract. The mechanism for this blood loss is not understood at the present time. You can also lose iron directly through sweat. In addition, exercise leads to a cascade of hormonal changes that end up reducing the iron levels in the blood by packing it away in storage sites. All of these mechanisms would be expected to reduce the amount of free, "bad" iron floating around in your body. Perhaps this is one reason why "a mile a day" is good for your heart.[17-19]

The "Iron Heart" Is a Weak One

In Chapter 7 you saw how iron can poison the hearts of iron-overload victims. As our understanding of heart disease continues to improve, it becomes apparent that excess iron may also be putting many other people at risk as well. The good news is that we can control our iron levels, attaining the lower iron levels of certain groups of people or societies in which heart disease is not epidemic. If you are not worried about any of the other scourges of Western societies, such as cancer, at least get iron-balanced for the sake of your heart.

10

Iron and Brain Disorders

The brain is the most important organ in the human body. It regulates our emotions, personality, intellect, physical movement, and involuntary bodily functions.

Brain disorders strike at the core of who we are. As our population ages, the number of people afflicted with various brain disorders will increase, and this will burden our already stressed health care system. In the hope of learning how to prevent the deterioration of brain function with age, the U.S. Congress has proclaimed the 1990s the Decade of the Brain. It is one of our final frontiers.

The links that have been established between iron and some brain diseases are provocative. Some of these links are stronger than others, but overall they should convince you that high iron levels are bad for your brain.

Stroke and You

Stroke is a sudden brain disorder caused by the interruption of the blood supply to a part of the brain. The symptoms, which depend on the part of the brain affected, include full or partial paralysis, altered vision or speech, the loss of sensation and of the ability to perceive the environment correctly, and various other patterns of weakness or sensory loss.

Up to half a million Americans each year suffer strokes. One in four victims dies within a month, making strokes the third leading cause of death in the U.S., after heart disease and cancer. Roughly two million Americans living today are disabled by strokes.

How can you reduce your risk of stroke? The recommendations commonly offered by doctors sound very much like those for preventing heart disease: lower your blood pressure and cholesterol level, don't smoke, and get some exercise. However, these measures seem to provide only partial protection. What more can we do to prevent strokes?

Iron and Stroke

In recent years there has been increasing interest in the role of iron in stroke. Since most strokes stem from a pattern of events similar to heart disease, including the gradual narrowing of arteries followed by brain-cell death after blood flow becomes blocked, many of the things you learned about iron in the previous chapter are applicable here. One possibility is that reducing our iron levels may slow the complex process involved in atherosclerosis, the disease of the arteries. A low-iron state could be healthy for the "pipes" in the brain, the heart, and perhaps the rest of the body as well.

The most important link between iron and stroke is in the process by which our vital brain cells die. Here again we have a parallel to coronary artery disease in that much of the damage is done not when blood flow is cut off but when it is resumed. The same sequence of events that results in the death of heart cells destroys brain cells, with iron playing a pivotal role.[1]

Animal studies have shown that the prior administration of an iron-binding drug that reduces iron availability can prevent the brain cells from self-destructing in simulated strokes. Other drugs that reduce the iron-induced damage are also being developed.

What about lowering our iron levels to prevent stroke and the damage that results from one? There is one provocative study, performed recently by Dr. John E. Repine and colleagues at the University of Colorado at Denver, that addressed this question.[2] The researchers fed one group of gerbils a low-iron diet for eight weeks. This led to lower blood and brain iron levels compared to those of animals fed a standard diet. The researchers then induced simulated strokes in the animals by clamping off one of the arteries supplying blood to the brain. After a few hours, the blood flow was restored, and the animals were observed for a period of time and then analyzed for brain damage. The low-iron animals fared much better than the control group in tests of brain function and tissue damage. While the results of these and other studies need to be confirmed in humans, they appear to be leading us into a new age of stroke prevention where the iron balance concepts may play an important role.

Parkinson's: The Shaking Disease

Let's consider another scourge of our elderly: neurodegenerative disease. This is a family of distinct conditions, many of which are commonly thought of as a natural part of aging. We are somewhat further from answers with regard to these diseases, including both their causes and optimal treatments, than we are with blood-flow-related disorders like stroke and coronary artery disease. The brain is an often enigmatic organ that reveals its secrets to researchers only very slowly. But research is progressing in this area, and we should see amazing progress in the 1990s.

One neurodegenerative disease with strong links to iron is Parkinson's disease, sometimes called shaking palsy. This condition, which usually begins in people between fifty and sixty-five years of age, presents a wide variety of different disabling symptoms, including the characteristic tremor as well as muscular rigidity and loss of balance. Other symptoms include diminished blinking, reduced spontaneity of facial expressions, and a tendency to remain in a single position for an unusually long period of time. It is usually the shaking tremor of the hands that brings most patients to a physician.

Parkinson's disease is extremely widespread, affecting over 400,000 Americans. Since many of its symptoms are often dismissed as stemming from old age, it has been estimated that as many as 40 percent of Parkinson victims may never get to a hospital and receive proper care.

The unique motion disorders in Parkinson's disease are known to stem from the destruction of cells in a small portion of the brain called the *substantia nigra.* Located strategically where the spinal cord meets the brain, the cells of the substantia nigra produce dopamine, a so-called neurotransmitter, which communicates signals to other parts of the brain that control complex movements. Patients are often treated successfully with L-dopa, a drug that is converted to dopamine in the brain, thus supplying what the Parkinson patient is lacking. However, large doses of L-dopa cause serious side effects, and many patients become unresponsive to the drug after about ten years. Research continues to determine the best way to treat victims whose brain cells are already destroyed.[3]

The real hope for the future, however, is in the prevention of Parkinson's disease. Scientists for some time have been trying to determine why these particular cells in the brain are dying. They have looked for environmental toxins, viruses, and other common causes of disease and have basically come up empty-handed.

Iron and Parkinson's Disease

The most recent evidence suggests that the enemy may be within, and that it might be iron. For unknown reasons, the cells in that critical region of the brain, the substantia nigra, accumulate a great deal of iron, even more than does the liver, a major iron-storing organ. Researchers have found that the iron content in this region of the brain in Parkinson patients is even higher than that found in unaffected people. One of the experts in this field, Dr. Moussa Youdim of the Israel Institute of Technology, has proposed that Parkinson's disease is a progressive disease involving iron-induced damage to this small and critical portion of the brain.[4] His theory has received wide recognition in recent years.

If the iron-Parkinson link stands the test of time and experimentation, scientists will have to address the following questions: by reducing our iron levels, can we decrease the amount of iron in our brains? If this does not work, can we prevent the accumulation of iron in the brain by maintaining low iron levels throughout life? Perhaps we will have the answers to these questions in the near future.

Alzheimer's Disease: A Path to Senility

Another neurodegenerative condition with even wider prevalence is Alzheimer's disease. The disease begins mildly with symptoms like forgetfulness, mood changes, and depression, often written off as the common effects of old age. Alzheimer's is indeed the major cause of senility. However, this condition leads to more serious effects as mental abilities continue to deteriorate. The victims become unable to work, lose their way in familiar surroundings, and often repeat conversations endlessly. Eventually the patients become completely incapacitated and dependent on others.

Alzheimer's disease is epidemic, with over 2.5 million people affected in the U.S. alone. The disease is thought to be responsible for 20 percent of the patients confined to nursing homes. And with our aging population, things will only get worse: by the year 2000, there could be over four million Alzheimer's victims.

We are even further behind in determining the cause and appropriate treatments for Alzheimer's disease than we are with Parkinson's. Scientists are focusing on odd clumps of protein both inside and outside the degenerating nerve cells. However, no clear answers have been forthcoming from this line of research. Investigators continue to look at other potential causes, such as defects in the immune system or inherited factors.

Aluminum, Iron, and Alzheimer's Disease

Another school of thought is that the development of Alzheimer's may be due to the accumulation of aluminum in the brain. Aluminum, a metallic substance with chemical properties similar to iron, is a common environmental pollutant.[5] A recent British government study showed that adults who consumed water with high concentrations of aluminum run a 50 percent greater risk of developing Alzheimer's than people whose water contains virtually no aluminum.[6] This study was important because aluminum has always been found in and around degenerating nerve cells. While some neuroscientists dismiss the aluminum as simply the effect of the disease, not the cause, other scientists continue to look more closely at the link between Alzheimer's, aluminum, and other metals like iron.

In a recent study published in the British journal *Lancet*, researchers found that the attachment of aluminum to proteins in the blood was somehow defective in Alzheimer's patients.[7] Since the binding of aluminum in the blood prevents the toxic metal from entering the brain, those people without this protective factor may suffer from aluminum accumulation in their brains for years, eventually resulting in neurological symptoms.

In addition to these findings, the study raised some interesting questions about iron levels in Alzheimer's patients. Although a larger number of patients would have to be studied for statistical significance, it did appear that the patients had higher iron levels than unaffected people. Since iron and aluminum attach to identical proteins in the blood, perhaps it was simply the high iron levels in Alzheimer's patients that displaced the aluminum from its safe sites in the blood, allowing it to enter the brain.

It is possible that the combination of high concentrations of *both* aluminum and iron in the brain is involved in this disease. For example, aluminum could kick iron out of safe storage sites and increase the amount of "bad" iron, which causes tissue damage. Some exciting, though preliminary, support for the importance of these metals in Alzheimer's disease comes from another recent *Lancet* study performed by Dr. Don R. C. McLachlan and co-workers at the University of Toronto.[8] In a three-year study, they found that desferrioxamine, the iron-binding drug that can also latch on to aluminum, could significantly reduce the mental degeneration caused by Alzheimer's.

As research in this area progresses, it may turn out that it's best to avoid iron and aluminum as much as possible. You can reduce your exposure to aluminum by avoiding aluminum cooking pots, aluminum-containing antacids and antiperspirants, and beverages in aluminum cans.

11

Iron and Cancer

Cancer is the disease many people fear the most. Though sometimes exaggerated, the horrible images of suffering from both the disease and the chemotherapy or radiation treatments are nonetheless imbedded in our minds. And the idea of our bodies attacking us from within is scary, to say the least.

As our population ages, cancer rates have been increasing. If you stay around long enough, your chances of getting some form of cancer are pretty good. It has been estimated that one in four of us will get some form of cancer during our lifetime. The disease is currently responsible for about 20 percent of all deaths in the U.S.; about one million new cases are reported each year.

The desire to prevent cancer by dietary and life-style changes has increased in recent years as scientists have begun to identify risk factors for the disease. While a great deal of effort has gone into understanding how environmental pollutants cause cancer, scientists are now finding that cancer is as likely to stem from within, from "natural" errors in cellular metabolism, as it is from external factors such as pesticides, other chemicals, or radiation. In a way this is good news, since we can often take positive steps to aid our internal defenses in this daily, mortal struggle against cancer.

As you will read in the pages that follow, iron has recently been identified as a risk factor for cancer. That iron, a "natural" and helpful element in our bodies, may have a dark side and may be involved in cancer fits well into recent trends in cancer research.

Cancer and Our Achilles' Heel

Though cancer really encompasses about a hundred different diseases depending on the tissue affected, the common denominator in each is the uncontrolled growth and spread of abnormal cells. The first step in getting these cells off on the wrong track is thought to be some form of chemical damage to our DNA, nature's sensitive Achilles' heel. This important substance, the cell's command control, is actually a long, chain link strand of four chemicals, the exact sequence of which forms the genetic code of life. Only a few changes in the sequence, even though it is billions of units in length, can cause a cell to grow out of control.

It is remarkable that most of us survive as long as we do without cancer taking us to an early grave. Scientists are finding that the DNA in each cell suffers over ten thousand "hits"— individual sites of chemical damage—every day.[1] Most of this daily scarring is caused by metabolic errors in our slightly less than perfect cellular machinery. Luckily, we possess a number of defense and repair troops. They furiously try to keep up with the damage. But now and then the damage is not repaired soon enough. Cancer may be the consequence.

Iron and Your DNA

While there are many chemicals that can cause DNA damage, the combination of iron and oxygen described in Chapter 2 is among the best at it. It has been known for many years that in the presence of oxygen, *iron is a carcinogen*, a cancer-causing chemical. Even the notorious carcinogenic properties of cigarette smoke and asbestos have been ascribed to the presence of iron. A lot of the early data in this field were based on the carcinogenic effects of relatively high concentrations of iron, such as the levels seen in iron-overload patients. However, identical chemical reactions can still take place, albeit at a slower rate, when moderately elevated levels of iron are present in the body.

The fact that iron is known to cause DNA damage has led some physicians, including Dr. William Crosby, director of hematology at the Chapman Cancer Center in Joplin, Missouri, and Dr. Margaret A. Krikker, president of the Hemochromatosis Research Foundation in Albany, New York, to question the legality of fortifying foods with this known carcinogen, even if it is a "natural substance" and even if it might help a small percentage of the population with iron deficiency.[2,3] Why take any chances?

Iron as "Food" for the Nasty Cancer Cell

A second way that iron may be involved in cancer is in stimulating the growth of tumor cells. While most of our normal cells have acquired a comfortable reserve of iron for their daily needs, new cancer cells are in serious need of iron if they are going to conquer their host. The cancer cell needs iron in order to divide and conquer, because the manufacture of DNA for the new cells involves a key iron-containing enzyme.

Dr. Baruch S. Blumberg, the author of the foreword to this book and one of the leaders in the area of iron-cancer links, has shown that tumors grow much more slowly in iron-deficient mice as compared to mice on a normal diet.[4] Conversely, other studies have shown that the administration of extra iron to mice with cancer leads to faster growth of the cancer cells and earlier death.[5]

You will be pleased to know that the body seems to know that iron is an important "food" for the cancer cells, and it reacts accordingly: it redirects iron to storage sites deep within certain organs, thus "starving" the cancer cells by decreasing the supply of available iron in the blood. This defense mechanism is also triggered when we become infected with bacteria or other microorganisms that try to divide and conquer within us. The false anemia that this iron-withholding defense causes was viewed negatively by doctors for many years. But over the past ten years iron experts such as Dr. Eugene Weinberg of Indiana University in Bloomington have begun to convince many that iron withholding and the mild anemia associated with it are beneficial to the patient.[6]

As is described further in Chapter 13, this iron-withholding defense is an indirect indication of how vital iron is to invading organisms and cancer cells. It is important that we do nothing to inhibit this natural response. When we are mildly iron-overloaded, as many of us are, this defense tactic is less effective.

Do Higher Iron Levels Result in Higher Cancer Rates?

A number of studies in the U.S. and abroad by Dr. Blumberg and other researchers have shown that high iron levels in people are associated with higher incidence of some forms of cancer.[7-10] These large population studies are often quite complex and difficult to interpret, and the conclusions from different studies often conflict. However, in every case where researchers examined iron explicitly, they have obtained evidence of the dangers of high iron levels.

The largest and most important of these studies was performed by Dr. Richard Stevens at the Battelle's Pacific Northwest Laboratories and his coworkers at the National Cancer Institute.[7] They examined data, including blood-iron measurements, from over 13,000 adults who were examined in detail as part of the First National Health and Nutrition Examination Survey (NHANES I). The appearance of cancer in these subjects was monitored for over ten years.

The results of this study, published in a 1988 issue of the *New England Journal of Medicine,* showed convincingly that men with higher iron levels were more likely to get some forms of cancer. This was especially true for cancer of the lungs, colon, esophagus (or throat), and bladder. As for women, the relationship between iron and cancer was less conclusive; however, the authors noted that women with the highest iron levels seemed to have higher cancer rates.

In addition to these studies, we also have evidence that iron causes cancer in patients with iron overload. As mentioned in Chapter 7, victims of hereditary hemochromatosis, compared to normal people, have two hundred times the risk of developing liver cancer.

Iron and the Cancer Prevention Diet

An interesting piece of indirect evidence for the iron-cancer link is that the American Cancer Society is now *inadvertently* recommending a diet that is fairly low in iron. The recommendations—less meat and more fruits, vegetables, and whole grains—are based on studies that revealed lower cancer risk for those populations who eat less fat and more fiber.[11] *But one reason why this diet might work is that it results in low iron absorption.*

In addition to the lower meat content, the inclusion of fiber is an important part of the recommended cancer prevention diet. The importance of a high-fiber diet stems largely from studies of colon cancer, which showed that those societies with more fiber in their diets enjoyed considerable protection from this form of cancer. The reasons for this protection are not entirely clear. Scientists thought that the undigested material in the intestines would aid bowel activity and decrease the amount of time the organ was exposed to potentially dangerous carcinogens in the diet. However, the importance of bowel transit time in colon cancer has been repeatedly questioned.[12-15]

Fiber and Phytic Acid

A new explanation of why a high-fiber diet protects against colon cancer has been offered by Dr. Ernst Graf of the Pillsbury Company and Dr. John Eaton of the University of Minnesota in

Minneapolis.[16] They proposed that perhaps it was not the un-digested fiber itself that was protective, but some other undi-gested plant substance. They focused on a substance called *phytic acid*, which is known to bind to iron strongly, preventing it from participating in dangerous chemical reactions.[17] If the iron in the bowel was bound up in this fashion, the interior of the intestine would suffer less chemical damage, and less iron would be ab-sorbed from the diet.

The phytic acid theory is supported by epidemiologic studies focused on diet and colon cancer. There is evidence that the intake of cereals, the high-fiber food with the most phytic acid, is responsible for the protective effect of high-fiber diets. Other high-fiber foods such as starch, vegetables, and fruits contain much lower amounts of phytic acid and were not found to be as important in preventing colon cancer.[18]

We will return to this topic in Chapters 16 and 17 and discuss how you can get more phytic acid in your diet.

All together, the available studies of iron and cancer confirm our more recent view of cancer: that it can often come from within rather than from external factors. Since there are many ways that a cell can go bad and turn cancerous, iron is likely to be only one of many factors. Just how important iron is com-pared to these other factors remains to be seen. For now, how-ever, it is easy to see that with the exception of quitting smoking, lowering our iron levels is as important as the other cancer-prevention steps that we may choose to take.

12

Iron and Aging

Aging is a process many of us know too well. It is as close to us as the back of our hands. Pinch the skin on the back of your hand for a few seconds and then let go. The longer it takes to snap back, the older you are. Gradual chemical changes within the skin cause it to become stiffer and less elastic, eventually leading to wrinkles, the common hallmark of aging.

While aging also results in other fairly benign changes, such as the graying of your hair and the increase in your golf score, it can also have much more serious effects, such as the weakening of the immune system that fights infection, gradual deterioration in hearing or sight, and the decline in functional efficiency of organs like the lungs, kidneys, and heart.

Aging, in addition to death and taxes, is part of being alive. It is a universal process in biology. Humans, mice, and even individual cells age, though they all differ in their rates of aging and expected life span. The maximum life span for a mouse is about three and a half years; for humans, it is 110–120 years. Scientists believe that there is not much we can do to increase these limits—they seem to be set by genetic factors. However, if we can slow the aging process somewhat, what we *can* do is push our individual life span closer to the maximum and enjoy life more along the way. To accomplish this we need to know more about the process underlying aging.

The leading theory of aging is that our cells become increasingly damaged by substances known as *free radicals,* toxic by-products of normal cellular processes. First proposed in 1954 by Dr. Denham Harman of the University of Nebraska College of Medicine in Omaha, the free-radical theory of aging has attracted increasing attention in recent years.[1] In support of the theory, scientists have found that cells are naturally equipped with protective enzymes that either detoxify the free radicals or correct the cellular damage the radicals inflict. Aging, as it turns out, results from the fact that these protective mechanisms simply cannot keep up with the damage. Depending on the targets within the cell that are hit, this damage can lead to deterioration in cell function, cell death, or, alternatively, to a loss in the control of the cell's growth, leading to cancer.

The Breath of Life Is Also the Breath of Death

The most toxic substances produced every day in our cells derive from the life-giving gas, oxygen. Most of the time oxygen is handled properly by the cell in the burning of fuel for cellular functions. However, now and then mistakes occur, and toxic oxygen by-products are released into the cell.

Many scientists now believe that the more oxygen an animal consumes in its resting state, the more of these toxic substances are produced. This in turn influences the aging rate and the maximum life span achievable. Mice, for example, consume much more oxygen per unit of body weight than humans and, as a result, they have much shorter life spans.

The lowly housefly has contributed to our understanding of the toxic effects of oxygen. Flies consume much more oxygen when flying than when they are at rest. If you clip the wings of houseflies or confine them to small containers, they consume much less oxygen and, remarkably, live significantly longer.[2,3]

Iron and Your Liver Spots

As you have read several times in this book, iron has a central role in the cellular mischief caused by oxygen by-products. The importance of iron in the aging process has only recently been recognized. Scientists have now determined that most of the cellular damage involves iron at some stage.

A role for iron has been established in one of the most fundamental processes of aging known today. This is the deposition in most tissues of a yellow-brown substance called *lipofuscin*, or *ceroid*. This substance, also known as age pigment, is one of the clearest signs of aging. Lipofuscin deposition often appears in the form of liver spots on the skin.[1,3]

Many scientists believe that lipofuscin results from the iron-assisted oxidation of cell walls and protein. Increasing the iron levels of both animals and people increases the amount of lipofuscin deposition. Thus iron directly increases the rate of a fundamental process involved in aging.[4,5]

There is an inherited disease where the accumulation of lipofuscin is abnormally rapid, and its victims show peculiar signs of premature aging. In this disease, known as *neuronal ceroid lipofuscinosis*, or NCL, massive accumulations of the pigment are seen throughout the nervous system, causing marked behavioral abnormalities, muscular and mental deterioration, and seizures. In terminal stages, patients adopt a contracted, fetal-like position and exhibit severe brain damage. Since elevated levels of iron have been found in the brain fluid of these patients, many scientists feel that this disease involves an abnormality of iron metabolism either as a cause or an effect.[3]

The Frail Male

If iron is involved in the fundamental process of aging itself, then we would expect that the gender difference in iron metabolism would affect aging and mortality rates. Indeed, you have already seen how higher iron levels in men may predispose them to heart disease, a major contributor to the gender gap in life expectancy. Men also die more frequently than women from a number of other ills such as cancer and various infectious diseases.

In assessing the vulnerability of males to many diseases, scientists have focused on various hormonal, genetic, and social factors. But they have ignored the "iron gap": a fundamental chemical difference between men and women that could be partly responsible for the relatively early deaths of men in our society.

Iron and Miscellaneous Diseases

Let us turn now to the wide range of conditions to which iron may contribute. One way to look for such diseases is to ask where scientists think oxygen free radicals are creating mischief. The list of such diseases has grown over recent years, and several medical conferences focused on oxygen-free-radical pathology have included discussions of sixty or more distinct conditions. These include disorders of the bowel (for example, inflammatory bowel disease), lungs (emphysema), eyes (cataracts), and kidneys (damage from cessation of blood flow).[2] However, at the time of this writing, direct effects of iron on these conditions have not been shown.

Clues From Iron-Overload Disease

A second way to look for diseases that may be influenced by iron levels is to closely examine those conditions associated with inherited iron-overload disease. Three common symptoms of iron overload are arthritis, liver disease, and sexual dysfunction. Perhaps moderately elevated iron levels can contribute to these conditions in normal (nonhemochromatotic) people.

Arthritis. In hemochromatosis, iron becomes deposited in the joints, which in turn leads to calcium deposits that can be seen on X rays of the knees and wrists. Similarly, iron is deposited in the joints of people inflicted by rheumatoid arthritis, the most severe form of arthritis, affecting five to eight million people in the U.S. The initial cause of the disease, in which the joints become inflamed, or swollen, and stiff, is unknown. However, the ongoing process of the disease is becoming better understood, and a definite role for iron has been discovered.

In rheumatoid arthritis, the synovial membrane, a sac that contains the lubricating fluid for the joint, becomes inflamed. A number of scientists, including arthritis expert Dr. David Blake at the London Hospital in England, believe that the joints of rheumatoid patients are degraded by the same form of iron-assisted oxidation that occurs in other diseases.[6] Iron, in particular, seems to be involved in the recurring flare-ups of the disease; these flare-ups are misread by the body, which reacts as if it is infected with bacteria or cancer cells and redistributes iron to certain locations, including the inflamed joint. Though the patients appear to be anemic on the basis of simple blood-iron levels, there is actually *more* iron in the worst possible place— in the joint itself—and this actually makes the disease worse. The whole cycle then begins to occur at more frequent intervals.

A number of observations have directly implicated iron in rheumatoid arthritis. In animal studies, for example, scientists have shown that true iron deficiency or the use of iron-sequestering drugs can significantly reduce the severity of the symptoms of rheumatoid arthritis. On the other hand, rheumatoid arthritis sufferers are often treated for the "false" anemia, which results from the body's response to the disease and the subsequent redistribution of iron. The supplemental iron often given to these patients essentially adds fuel to the fire and exacerbates the disease.[6] If you have rheumatoid arthritis, you should be very careful about increasing the iron content of your diet.

Alcohol and Liver Disease. As you read in Chapter 7, liver disease is one of the most important signs of iron overload. In some cases, doctors have mistaken the liver disease of iron overload with that stemming from a more common toxin, alcohol. As it turns out, the effects of these two toxins may be interrelated. Scientists are finding that alcohol-induced liver damage involves, like so many other diseases, that familiar deadly duo of iron and oxygen. Just as alcohol can exacerbate the liver damage in hemochromatosis victims, elevated iron levels in drinkers can predispose them to greater liver damage. This is discussed further in Chapter 17.

Sexual Dysfunction. Along with arthritis and liver disease, sexual dysfunction is another common sign of iron overload. Hemochromatosis apparently leads to iron accumulation in the pituitary gland of the brain, and this, in turn, interferes with the proper secretion of sex hormones. This results in decreased sexual desire for both sexes and diminution in the size of the testes and impotence in males.

Could moderately elevated iron levels also reduce sexual capability or desire? Unfortunately, we do not yet know the answer to this question. However, we do know that our brains accumulate iron as we age, and it is reasonable to expect that the critical pituitary gland would not be spared in this general "rusting" process. Though the brain iron levels due to aging are not expected to be as high as those in hemochromatosis patients, even a moderate excess, especially over long periods of time, could lead to pituitary damage. Clearly, the safest bet to preserve our sexual capability would be to keep our iron levels low throughout life.

Iron and Your Appearance

Finally, let's get back to where we started in this chapter: your skin. Will living a low-iron life-style help your skin stay young? While we have no direct evidence at this point about whether or not changes in iron levels will affect this active and complex organ, the term *oxygen free radicals* is popping up all over the current issues of dermatology journals. Iron should be close behind.

Keeping iron levels low could reduce the number or density of liver spots, those yellow-brown areas containing lipofuscin, the aging pigment.

How about wrinkling? This is something we would all like to prevent. Free radicals are thought to be at work in both the normal aging of skin as well as that caused by the sun, which is known as photo-aging. Wrinkling is thought to be caused by chemical changes to important structural proteins in the skin. The aging-related damage in these proteins can be produced in a test tube with that familiar and dangerous combination of iron and oxygen.

Another dermatological condition in which free radicals have been implicated is dandruff, which results from the oxidation of scalp cells. Many substances that slow this process, for example those found in some dandruff shampoos, are known to slow the oxidation process.[7] A similar effect would be expected with lower iron levels, though this has not been directly tested.

13

The Iron-Depletion Hypothesis: Less Is Best

From the preceding chapters, I think you can see that lately there has been a lot of bad press on iron. This nutrient had an excellent public relations campaign going for a long time, but it has fooled us long enough. From our outsides to our insides, from our skin to our hearts, iron is at work in harmful ways. You can now see that we do not have to stretch that Kipling allegory in Chapter 1 too far: iron is indeed a slave ring around our necks. Our health is the hostage.

The Central Concept Behind the Iron Balance Health Plan

In response to the growing evidence that excess iron is bad for us, several scientists have begun to support a radical redefinition of the proper amount of iron that should be in our bodies. This group of scientists, which includes Dr. Baruch Blumberg of the Fox Chase Cancer Center, Dr. Jerome Sullivan of the Medical University of South Carolina, Dr. Eugene Weinberg of Indiana

University, Dr. Richard Stevens of Battelle's Pacific Northwest Laboratories, and others mentioned in previous chapters, has questioned the conventional definition of the "normal" and healthy iron levels in humans.[1-4] Their own proposal, often referred to as the iron-depletion hypothesis, states that if we deplete our bodies of excess storage iron, we will enjoy lower incidence of certain diseases. This concept is the basis of the Iron Balance Health Plan.

Let's briefly examine the logic behind this important redefinition of optimal iron levels. First, we should no longer view the accumulation of large amounts of storage iron as a natural and healthy process. Many of us accumulate a gram or so of this form of iron as we age, more than we can ever utilize. All of this excess rust is certainly not doing us any good. While our iron stores should be sufficient to make up for day-to-day variations in iron intake and loss, they should not be excessive.

Second, low iron stores may permit the earlier detection of certain serious illnesses. Many common diseases, including colon cancer and ulcers, cause blood loss that is hidden in the stool. The replacement of lost red blood cells requires iron from the body's reserves. If you have one of these conditions and your iron stores are comfortably low, you will quickly develop a mild anemia, which your doctor can detect with routine blood tests. With high iron stores, it may be years before you develop the telltale anemia, and the disease at that point is likely to be more advanced and more difficult to treat.

Finally, the most important benefit of the low-iron state is the reduced incidence of certain diseases. It appears that the amount of "bad" iron, iron that is not bound to protective proteins, increases as we accumulate excessive iron stores. This "bad" form of iron can either initiate tissue damage or contribute to disease processes.

Iron Depletion Is Natural

The human body seems to know all this: iron depletion is a *natural* defense mechanism used by the body to fight infection and cancer. As part of a complex set of responses to infectious bacteria and tumor cells, your body tries to starve them of the iron they need to grow by diverting the metal from the blood to storage sites deep within the tissues. The body's response to the invasion of such organisms is rapid and profound, with serum iron levels dropping to 30 percent of normal values.

The drop in iron levels during infection has been recognized for years but has often been viewed negatively by the medical community. The term "anemia of chronic disease" is often applied to this effect, perpetuating the notion that it is detrimental to the health of the patient, when in fact it is beneficial. Experts in this area, such as Dr. Eugene Weinberg, have pointed out how important this iron-withholding defense is to the patient in fighting infection.[5,6]

If your body is high in iron, this defense mechanism is not as effective. Sometimes physicians have treated people with this anemia of chronic disease by prescribing iron supplements; in many cases, this actually exacerbates the infection by providing iron to the virulent organisms. This is the reason, according to the old adage, you are supposed to "starve a fever." In addition to the diversion of iron in the body, the rise in body temperature that follows infection reduces the iron-scavenging ability of bacteria. Eating a lot of iron-rich foods would counter both defenses.

The incidence of some forms of infections and cancer is known to be lower in societies where people have low iron levels, such as in developing countries. There is even a theory that fewer women than men died from the horrible Black Plague of medieval Europe because of their lower iron levels.[7]

This natural mechanism to protect us from microbial invasion seems to be telling us something: perhaps it is more "natural" to have low iron levels. During evolution, humans and other animals had a difficult time getting too much iron because food was scarce. In Western societies today, however, most of us *do* get too much iron, from fortified foods and high meat intake. And the human body unfortunately has no way to get rid of excess iron. The bounteous life-style overwhelms a body designed for leaner times.

How Low Should Our Iron Levels Be?

Take a look at Figure 13-1 to review what you learned about iron accumulation in Chapter 2. You will remember that premenopausal, menstruating women have the lowest iron levels: about 100–400 milligrams of stored iron. Men and postmenopausal women, on the other hand, lack the regular blood-loss mechanism of menstruation and quickly build up dangerous levels of iron, up to 1000 milligrams or even 1500 milligrams or more.

Though it is difficult at this early stage to predict the safest iron level—and it may vary from person to person—it is likely that the levels of 100–400 milligrams, comparable to those of most younger women, is best. This is a comfortable reserve of iron to meet the day-to-day variations in iron intake and loss. More important, this relatively low level of iron seems to be an

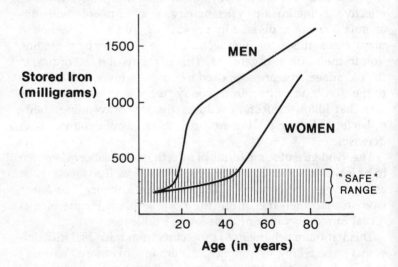

Figure 13-1. The iron levels of most men and older women are excessive. This is a plot of the average iron stores in men and women as a function of age. The optimal level of iron that provides a comfortable reserve without being excessive is shown as the "safe" range of 100–400 milligrams. While most premenopausal women have iron levels within this optimal range, most men and older women exceed this level by up to 1000 milligrams or more.

important factor in the protection from heart disease that younger women enjoy. This "safe" range is shown in Figure 13-1. You can see how much excess iron many of us have to lose to get into this optimal range.

We should not try to adjust our iron levels much below 100–400 milligrams, since it could lead to anemia. Severe anemia is a serious medical condition requiring the attention of a physician. (See Chapter 15 for more on this.) Mild anemia, on the other hand, is less of a problem. As discussed in Chapter 5, the only demonstrated negative effects of mild anemia are on *peak* work or exercise performance. If you are not a professional athlete or manual laborer, you do not need to worry about this. Few of us work or exercise at the extremely high levels where mild anemia can have an effect. Nonetheless, one should still shoot for a sufficient reserve of at least 100 milligrams of storage iron. The following chapters will show you how to reach and maintain an optimum iron level.

The Future of Iron Depletion, and You

It is important to point out that, though the evidence is clear for some diseases, the iron-depletion hypothesis, like any other theory, must be tested in each case. Absolute scientific proof always requires extensive, controlled clinical trials. Disease incidence in thousands of matched subjects, some with low iron levels and some without, will be studied for up to ten years or even longer. The results from different trials will be subject to rigid statistical analysis, and in the end, they may give conflicting results because of the choice of subjects, biological variability, and so on. To see the unavoidable problems that scientists encounter in this process, one only has to look at the confusion that now exists in properly defining the value of lowering cholesterol in preventing coronary artery disease. Cholesterol's role has been known for years, yet questions still remain.

Because the links between moderate levels of iron and disease are just now surfacing, you can imagine how long the road to absolute certainty is going to be. In addition, many in the medical establishment will fight against the iron-depletion theory. The notions that iron is only a "do-good" nutrient and that millions of women still do not get enough iron are firmly ingrained in the minds of thousands of doctors. Will they do an about-face on this topic when the early data on the dangers of iron become widely discussed? Hardly.

The evidence we have now is, I believe, more than sufficient for us to begin to practice the safe preventative measures that form the core of the Iron Balance Health Plan. I will describe these steps in the following how-to chapters.

Part 5

THE IRON BALANCE HEALTH PLAN

14

The Iron-Risk-Level Self-Test

What do all these revelations about iron mean for your health? How can you become iron-balanced and maximize your chances for a long and healthy life?

The rest of this book gives you the answer to these questions: the Iron Balance program. This new health plan shows you how to reduce the amount of excess iron in your body and maintain a low but more than adequate level of stored iron for life.

But first, you need an idea of where you are starting out: how much excess iron do you have stored away in your body?

Where Do You Stand Today?

In reading the earlier chapters, you may have been thinking, "I took iron-containing supplements for several years. I wonder what this did to my iron level?" If you eat a lot of iron-rich meat, or if you are a woman who has taken oral contraceptives, which reduce menstrual blood loss, you may be wondering how these factors have affected your iron level. On the other hand, you may have decreased the amount of excess iron in your body if you have donated blood recently. But the question still remains: how much has this lowered your risk of iron-related diseases?

The Iron-Risk-Level Self-Test gives you an estimate of where you stand today with respect to true iron balance. All that is required is a pencil and a few minutes of your time. The score that you compute, which crudely approximates the amount of stored iron in your body, can be compared to average values for your age and sex and to the individual scores for various people, including the author.

Please keep in mind that by simply answering a few questions there is absolutely no way that the *actual* amount of iron in your body can be calculated accurately. The Iron-Risk-Level Self-Test is only a very crude way of doing this. It is good at delivering an answer quickly, so that you get some idea of where you stand right now. But it in no way substitutes for an actual iron-status measurement, which your doctor can perform. Obtaining a serum ferritin measurement, which is described further in Chapter 2, is a recommended step in the Iron Balance program (see Chapter 20). The serum ferritin test, which requires only a couple tablespoons of your blood, is a fairly accurate measurement of stored iron.

How does your Iron-Risk-Level Self-Test score relate to the more accurate blood test? Scientists have found that if you multiply the number reported in a serum ferritin measurement by ten, the resulting product is usually a good approximation of the total amount of stored iron in the body:

$$\underline{\hspace{2cm}} \quad \times \quad 10 \quad = \quad \underline{\hspace{2cm}}$$

Serum Ferritin Measurement From Your Doctor (in units of micrograms per liter or nanograms per milliliter)	Estimated Amount of Stored Iron (in milligrams)

For example, a serum ferritin level of 100 units indicates a total iron load of 1000 milligrams. The Iron-Risk-Level Self-Test estimates this same value—the amount of stored iron—in the same units, milligrams. If you are curious to see how accurate your Iron-Risk-Level Self-Test score is, you can directly compare it to the ferritin test results after multiplying the latter by ten as described above.

While the Iron-Risk-Level Self-Test is only a crude estimate of iron status, the mere process of taking the test gives you an immediate picture of just how important different factors are in determining your iron-risk level. For example, which is worse: eating a lot of meat or taking iron supplements? Just how much of an effect do oral contraceptives have on iron levels? Which is better for decreasing iron levels, blood donation or exercise? The Iron-Risk-Level Self-Test is scientifically designed to properly weigh each one of these factors.

The Iron-Risk-Level Self-Test has five simple steps. In step 1, you select a baseline value of your iron-risk level appropriate for your age and sex. This value is numerically equal to the estimated average amount of stored iron (in milligrams) for people in your population subgroup (see Figure 2-1 in Chapter 2). In the following steps you adjust your score by adding or subtracting different quantities of iron depending on your life-style and habits.

In steps 2 and 3, you add to your baseline number if you take iron-containing supplements or if you fall into certain categories of premenopausal women.

In step 4, you either add to or subtract from the number you got in step 3 depending on the average number of servings of meat you eat each day. Vegetarians will reduce their iron-risk level score, whereas avid carnivores will increase it.

In the final step, step 5, you may get to reduce your score if you have donated blood recently or if you exercise regularly. The final result is your iron-risk level score.

The Iron-Risk-Level Self-Test

Step 1. Choose your Baseline Score from the following table:

WOMEN		MEN	
Age (in years)	*Baseline Score*	*Age (in years)*	*Baseline Score*
under 18	210	under 18	230
18–30	240	18–20	380
31–40	280	21–22	690
41–50	370	23–30	930
51–60	630	31–40	1040
61–70	960	41–50	1180
over 70	1250	51–60	1310
		61–70	1420
		over 70	1560

Your Baseline Score
(in milligrams of stored iron)

Step 2. Do you consume iron-containing supplements or highly fortified cereal products? If so, and if these contain 18 milligrams of iron (100 percent of the current U.S. RDA) or more, add one of the following quantities to your baseline score:

If you have been consuming such products approximately 2–4 times per week for:

	add:
6 months	+ 60
1 year	+120
1.5 years	+180
2 or more years	+240

If you have been consuming such products five times per week or more for:

	add:
6 months	+120
1 year	+240
1.5 years	+360
2 or more years	+480

If you do not consume such products, enter zero.

_____   +   _____   =   _____
Baseline Score   Iron-Supplement   Step-2 Score
(from step 1)   Score

Step 3. If you are a premenopausal woman, add to the step-2 score if you fall into either (or both) of these categories:
If you have been taking oral contraceptives for:

	add:
1 year	+ 38
2 years	+ 75
3 years	+113
4 or more years	+150

If you have *not* been menstruating regularly for:

	add:
6 months	+110
1 year	+220
1.5 years	+330
2 years	+440
2.5 years	+550
3 or more years	+660

If you are a premenopausal woman who does not fall into either of these two categories, or if you are a man or postmenopausal woman, enter zero.

_____	+	_____	+	_____	=	_____
Step-2 Score		Oral Contraceptive Score		Amenorrhea Score		Step-3 Score

Step 4. If you eat two or more servings of meat, fish, or poultry on average each day, add the appropriate quantity to the step-3 score. (One serving of meat is generally three ounces, a little larger than a regular McDonald's hamburger patty. If your average serving sizes are significantly larger than this, use the estimate of 1.5 or 2 servings per meal.)

amount of meat per day
(for 1 year or more)   *add:*
2 servings   + 240
2.5 servings   + 480
3 or more servings   + 720

_____	+	_____	=	_____
Step-3 Score		Heavy-Meat-Eater Score		Step-4 Score

If you eat only about 1.5 servings of meat, fish, or poultry each day (in other words, sometimes one serving per day, sometimes two), then add nothing to your step-3 score:

_____	+	0	=	_____
Step-3 Score		Moderate-Meat-Eater Score		Step-4 Score

If you are a total vegetarian or eat only a little meat each day, then *subtract* the appropriate quantity from your step-3 score (if the result is a negative answer, just enter zero):

amount of meat per day
(for 1 year or more)   subtract:
              0 serving   370
              0.5 serving   305
              1 serving   240

_____ – _____ < = _____

Step-3 Score   Light-Meat-Eater   Step-4 Score
                      Score

Step 5. If you have donated blood in the last year or two, and/ or if you are currently exercising regularly, *subtract* the following quantities from your step-4 score:

number of blood donations (1 pint)
         in last year or two   subtract:
                    1   200
                    2   400
                    3   600
              4 or more   800

amount of aerobic exercise
(20 minutes or more)
practiced for a year or   subtract:
         more
3–5 times a week   50
6 or 7 times a week   100
athletic training   200

_____ – _____ – _____ = _____

Step-4   Blood   Exercise   Total Iron-Risk-
Score   Donation   Score   Level Score
           Score   (in milligrams
                                          of
                                     stored iron)

How Do You Rank?

Your iron-risk-level score places you in one of four risk levels. The categories listed below are in the order of increasing probability that iron could contribute to adverse health effects.

1. *Low Risk:* A score of 0–400 milligrams of stored iron. This is the "safe" range of iron values, as represented by premenopausal women, who exhibit lower rates of several chronic diseases, especially heart disease. If you scored in this range, that's good! You may already be iron-balanced! But keep in mind that the score is only a rough estimate of your iron load: it could underestimate the actual value. You also need to keep in mind that any biological events, such as menopause for women, or significant life-style changes could quickly increase your iron risk. Thus, even if your score is correct, you should read the remainder of this book to identify exactly what it is that you are doing right. This will go a long way toward keeping you iron-balanced for life.

2. *Intermediate Risk:* A score of 400–800 milligrams of stored iron. If you scored in this range, you are not doing too badly, but you may need to reduce your iron level by following the Iron Balance plan. It is difficult to say whether people in this zone (mostly women) would exhibit any adverse health consequences due to iron. Nonetheless, the low-risk category is safest, and you should strive to get there.

3. *High Risk:* A score of 800–1600 milligrams of stored iron. This is a broad range that includes most men and older postmenopausal women (over sixty years of age). The high-risk nature of this group is illustrated by their greater risk of heart attacks as compared to premenopausal women. If you scored in this range, ask yourself, "Why do I need all this excess, useless, and potentially dangerous iron?" You should take a closer look at your "high-iron habits" and start trimming your iron level today.

4. *Very High Risk:* A score of greater than 1600 milligrams of stored iron. If you scored this high, you are probably a heavy meat-eater and/or you have been needlessly taking iron supplements or eating highly fortified cereals. These are serious "high-iron habits" that you need to stop. It may take you a little longer to get iron-balanced, but you can get there.

How Does Your Score Compare to Others?

Let's take a look at four men and four women and see how they score on the Iron-Risk-Level Self-Test. A few of these people really exist, though their real names are not used, but most are composites of more than one person.

Randall, age thirty-two. Self-test score: 800 milligrams. As you may have guessed, this is my test score from 1989. The score reported here is for the period prior to my beginning the Iron Balance program. My baseline score was 1040, and the only adjustment to this was a subtraction of 240 due to fairly light meat consumption, about a serving per day, usually at dinner. Since I occasionally ate meat for lunch, you could say that my true score was probably a little higher than 800. Thus, I categorize my pre–Iron Balance self as being at the lower end of the high-risk level, which encompasses most male omnivores like myself.

In my case, I got a serum ferritin test before beginning the Iron Balance program. Multiplying the test result, 88 units, by ten gave me an estimate of 880 milligrams of stored iron in my body, not far from the self-test result of 800 milligrams or so. In Chapter 20, I will show you how both my serum ferritin values and my self-test scores dropped in unison when I began the Iron Balance program.

Bill, age forty-five. Self-test score: 875 milligrams. Bill joins me at the lower end of the high-risk range. He was able to subtract 305 from his baseline score of 1180 since he eats only about half a serving of meat a day. (His wife is a complete vegetarian; he is only a partial convert.) Despite his light meat consumption, he still needs to reduce his iron level.

Tom, age fifty-five. Self-test score: 1790 milligrams. With large servings of meat usually at both lunch (cheese-steak subs, quarter-pound hamburgers) and dinner (steaks and roasts), Tom joins other "meat-and-potatoes" guys in the very-high-risk category. His estimate of 2.5 servings of meat per day (due to the large servings he eats at lunch and dinner) forced him to add 480 to his baseline score of 1310. Men like Tom often have the worst possible combination: high iron *and* high cholesterol levels. They might as well put out the welcome mat for a heart attack.

Richard, age fifty-three. Self-test score: 1340 milligrams. Richard has a similar occupation and diet to Tom but works for a different company. Within the last couple of years, a local hospital came around twice with the "bloodmobile" and asked the employees to donate. Richard donated both times and, as a result, was able to decrease his self-test score by 400. He also exercises 3–5 times a week, permitting another 50-milligram deduction. This placed Richard in the high-risk category—still bad, but not nearly as dangerous as the level that Tom is at.

Ann, age twenty-nine. Self-test score: 280 milligrams. Ann is your typical, premenopausal Jane Doe. She eats meat at dinner and at about half of her lunches (1.5 servings per day) and takes no iron-containing supplements or oral contraceptives. Her baseline score is her final score, and she is clearly in the low-risk category. She is in perfect iron balance.

Debbie, age thirty. Self-test score: 670 milligrams. For more than two years, two to four times a week, Debbie, unlike Ann, has been taking a multivitamin-mineral supplement containing 100 percent of the RDA for iron. She read in a women's magazine that women need more iron, so she chose the iron-containing supplement over another product made by the same company that contains no iron. Debbie has also been taking oral contraceptives for more than four years. These two seemingly innocent life-style differences raised Debbie's score a total of 390 milligrams above Ann's and put Debbie in the intermediate-risk category.

Margaret, age fifty-five. Self-test score: 870 milligrams. Margaret, like many postmenopausal women, joins myself and Bill, both younger males, at the lower end of the high-risk range. She has lost that important protective factor, menstruation, and she has not modified her life-style to compensate for the loss. Like Tom, her husband, she continues to eat two servings of meat a day, and like most people, she does not know how to lower her iron levels through exercise and blood donation. Her risk of having a heart attack, like that of most postmenopausal women, is rapidly increasing with age.

Elizabeth, age 70. Self-test score: 1200 milligrams. Like most senior citizens, men and women, Elizabeth is in a high-risk category. To keep her cholesterol level down and to prevent cancer, she has reduced her meat intake to one serving per day. This gives her a 240-point deduction from her baseline score of 960. However, she unknowingly counteracts this healthy measure by taking a popular iron supplement in liquid form, believing it will increase her energy and stamina. Since she has been taking this supplement almost every day for over two years, she must add 480 points to her score, placing her in the middle of the high-risk category. While it is good for her to keep her fat and cholesterol intake low, the excess iron in her system could contribute to health problems in the future.

Your Score and Your Actual Iron Stores

As described, the Iron-Risk-Level Self-Test was pretty good at approximating my own experimentally measured iron level. For many people, however, the self-test is far too simple to pinpoint iron levels. What might lead the test to give a result that is way off the actual value?

Let's deal first with a case where the self-test gives a low estimate of iron stores. One important way in which this may occur is if you have either the mild or full-blown form of hemochromatosis, the inherited disease in which too much iron is absorbed in the intestines (see Chapter 7). Your actual iron level—and that of your blood relatives—could be very high with this disease. This could lead eventually to several adverse health effects, particularly in the case of the full-blown form of the disease.

Another situation in which the self-test estimate is too low is if you had taken iron supplements years ago. Since it is difficult to take this into account, the self-test focuses on recent years and thus might not account for some buildup of iron stores. This could occur after pregnancy, for example, if high doses of iron supplements are consumed for long periods.

On the other hand, your self-test results might be too high if you had suffered considerable blood loss, and therefore iron loss, at some point in your life. This might occur from an accident, surgery, pregnancy, heavy menstruation, or a chronic condition such as an ulcer or colon cancer. Without iron supplementation, these events can significantly reduce the amount of storage iron.

As part of the Iron Balance program, I urge you to get a full iron analysis from your doctor within the first year. Then you will know for sure if the self-test is giving you a false sense of security or a false alarm.

A Word on Medical Risk

To further place your self-test score and even your iron level as measured by your doctor in the proper perspective, you need to appreciate just how much medicine is still an art in this age of science. Doctors can often predict what percentage of a given population will get a particular disease, but they can't tell you whether *you'll* get it. The odds for correctly predicting any one individual's fate are about the same as for winning at roulette.

Often the best your doctor can do is tell you whether you are "at risk" for the disease. For example, if your blood-cholesterol level is 260—that is, 260 milligrams per deciliter of blood—your doctor will say that you are among the 10 percent of the population with the highest cholesterol, and that these individuals historically suffer a somewhat higher rate of heart attacks than those at lower levels. But plenty of people with cholesterol readings of 220 still get the disease. Therefore, cholesterol is a rather "soft" risk factor for coronary artery disease: no clear cutoff value between high- and low-risk patients exists.

Since the iron story is still developing, we do not know where it stands relative to cholesterol as a risk factor for disease. Will it be "hard" or "soft"? Will combination indices, such as the iron-cholesterol index described in Chapter 9, be better at separating high- and low-risk patients? While scientists are busy sorting this out, I am going to cover my bets and get iron-balanced in any case.

15

Iron Balance for Women and Children

The vast majority of adult males in our society have accumulated potentially dangerous amounts of iron in their bodies. Men in general can—and should—practice the Iron Balance Health Plan vigorously and need not be concerned about becoming anemic.

However, the same generalization cannot be made for children and certain categories of women. Pregnant women require substantial amounts of iron for the proper growth of the fetus. The same goes for children during their growth years. Women also have a small chance of becoming anemic due to excessive menstrual flow or low iron intake in weight-loss diets. While postmenopausal women can jump into the Iron Balance program wholeheartedly, younger women and children must exercise caution.

This chapter outlines special concerns regarding iron balance for these groups of people.

Women and the Iron Story

Women hold a special place in the iron story. The discovery of the importance of nutritional iron stemmed largely from observations of the pale, tired faces of young, iron-deficient women years ago. The prevalence of iron-deficiency anemia in women today, however, has been exaggerated. Indeed, iron deficiency has become one of the most overdiagnosed conditions in America. In the latter half of the twentieth century, women have become targets of companies selling iron supplements, when in fact most of these women have sufficient iron stores. For the legions of tired women, often juggling homemaking, motherhood, and a career, the cause of their fatigue lies elsewhere.

Premenopausal women, in particular, are important to consider because they comprise the largest segment of the population that is at least close to being truly iron-balanced. For most of these women, their nutritional intake of iron appears to balance their losses, and they do not accumulate the excessive iron stores that men do.

It appears to be just one more example of bias in our male-dominated medical establishment that the low iron stores in menstruating women are seen as insufficient, unhealthy, or dangerous. The mind-set of physicians has been, "A normal man has over a gram of storage iron in his body; why shouldn't a woman?" Armed with our new iron facts, we need to turn the tables on this type of logic and instead of asking what is wrong with the women, ask what is wrong with the men.

Perhaps part of the problem in defining the proper amount of storage iron lies in the long-running neglect of women's health problems by the medical establishment. John Doe, aged forty-five to sixty-four, has been studied intensively to find risk factors for heart disease and other conditions. There are many cries in the media now that Jane Doe needs to be studied in as much detail. Perhaps if we had been doing this all along, we would have seen more clearly how women's bodies appear to protect them from some diseases, rather than just seeing what is going wrong in men's bodies.

A New View of Menstruation

That intensely private, sometimes troubling, but natural physiological process we call menstruation is largely what separates women from men with regard to iron levels. The rhythmical loss of iron through roughly half a woman's lifetime keeps her iron stores in check. There is good evidence that low iron levels reduce the incidence of some diseases in women. A good example is that of heart disease, where, as you read in Chapter 9, a woman's protection seems to be based not on hormones but on the lower iron levels she is able to maintain due to the regular blood loss of menstruation.

Once again, it is possible our belated realization of the importance of menstruation to overall health is due to entrenched ideas. The concept that menstruation itself, or any other form of bleeding for that matter, has direct health benefits is as alien to today's physicians as the idea that the earth orbits the sun was to Copernicus's contemporaries. While the medical establishment would prefer to express their objections to these ideas using cold, hard, scientific reasoning, one cannot help but think that society's squeamishness about menstruation, particularly on the part of men, may have played a role. These attitudes, along with a dose of male chauvinism, may also be responsible in part for the neglect that "women's problems" have suffered until recently. These important medical problems include the physiological and psychological effects of both menstruation and menopause.

The roots of our fears or unease concerning menstruation run deep into our heritage. In ancient cultures the strange monthly bleedings left men in awe and in fear. There had to be something supernatural about women, for how else could they survive? Men could not see the link with a woman's procreative abilities and instead viewed the process as unclean, or much worse, as evil. To protect the crops and the village, women in many primitive cultures were banished to special huts during menstruation. In ancient Persia, this isolation was accompanied by lashes to remove the evil spirit. In more forgiving cultures, women were to signal their condition to others. If a Congo woman was greeted by a man on a day when she was menstruating, she could pop a pipe in her mouth as a sign that she could not answer because she was "unclean."

The taboos about menstruation continued in one form or another in the development of religions and in our present-day culture. A classic example from today is the "religious truth" about menstruation as told by the ingenuous Archie Bunker in the television series *All in the Family:*

> Read your Bible. Read about Adam and Eve. . . . Going against direct orders, she makes poor Adam take a bite out of that apple. So God got sore and told them to get their clothes on and get outta there. So, it was Eve's fault God cursed women with this trouble. That's why they call it, what do you call it, the curse.

Society's squeamishness was evident in the flood of critical mail received by the writers of this television episode complaining about the use of the word *menstruation* in the script. (Even the technical term *menstruation* is euphemistic: rather than "monthly bleeding," it is merely Latin for "monthly.")[1]

One hopes these views will change. Menstruation is not unclean or unhealthy. It is not "the weeping of a disappointed uterus." It is not a female flaw or weakness. It is just part of a natural and beautiful rhythm of nature that prepares a woman for the creation of new life. To this we can add the heretofore hidden knowledge that, with today's high-iron life-style, menstruation actually has important health benefits in preventing excessive iron buildup. Menstruation should be viewed not as a curse but as a blessing, though sometimes an inconvenient one.

Losing the Menstrual "Blessing"

If we average the amount of iron lost through each menstrual period over the entire month, it comes out to about half a milligram per day. When menstruation ceases or is reduced in intensity, iron is largely retained by the body, and it accumulates with time in the same way it does in men. Whether or not anyone might suffer any adverse health consequences from this iron accumulation depends largely on how long it persists.

Let's look at three situations where this occurs:

Menopause. Along with the hot flashes, increased risk of osteoporosis, and the psychological consequences of menopause, we must now include the added health risk of iron accumulation. At menopause, a woman's iron level begins to climb, approaching that of a man's. The propensity for heart disease, that deadly trait of manhood, follows closely. It is also possible that the increased risk of infections that accompanies menopause could be in part due to or exacerbated by higher iron levels; bacteria and yeast, held in check by the lack of freely available iron, could thrive more easily if the iron supply increases.

If you are a woman in her mature years, the Iron Balance program is for you.

Amenorrhea. The loss of regular periods should always be brought to the attention of a doctor. This can be due to excessive dieting or exercise, as well as pregnancy, minor hormonal disturbances, or more serious problems related to the pituitary or thyroid gland, disturbances of the nervous system or ovaries, anorexia nervosa, or other psychological disorders or illnesses.

Whether or not you need to be concerned about iron buildup during amenorrhea depends on the length of time it persists. If it is only temporary or it responds promptly to drugs or changes in behavior, then you may not need to be too concerned. You should still have a full iron work-up by your doctor, as recommended in Chapter 20. But in general, as a young or middle-aged woman, you are most likely fairly close to being iron-balanced.

If, on the other hand, this is a chronic condition, there is no doubt that you are at risk of building up excess iron in your tissues. Follow the Iron Balance recommendations closely.

It is also important to keep in mind that amenorrhea has been seen as a presenting symptom of hemochromatosis, the hereditary iron-overload disease discussed in Chapter 7. Iron in the pituitary gland destroys the proper secretions of hormones. If your family has any history of liver disease, congestive heart failure, diabetes, or hormonal imbalances, you and your relatives should be screened for this inherited disease. This screening test is an integral part of the Iron Balance program (see Chapter 20).

Oral Contraceptives. Taking oral contraceptives has certain advantages, such as effective and convenient birth control and regular, predictable, and light periods. This latter advantage of low menstrual flow is actually a disadvantage when viewed from the perspective of iron balance. Oral contraceptives decrease menstrual blood loss to a third or half that of women who do not take them. With lower iron losses, you are more likely to accumulate iron.

A 1985 study of the effect of oral contraceptives on iron status in women confirmed that taking oral contraceptives for two or more years does indeed increase the amount of excess iron stored in the body. Using serum ferritin measurements, Erica Frassinelli-Gunderson and colleagues at the University of California at Berkeley found that forty-six women taking oral contraceptives had larger amounts of stored iron (an average of approximately 400 milligrams) than seventy-one women who did not take them (an average of around 200 milligrams).[2]

This side effect of oral contraceptives has always been overlooked by the medical community. The increase in iron levels could contribute to the increased heart disease risk in those who use oral contraceptives, particularly women who smoke cigarettes. Furthermore, like menopausal women, users could be more susceptible to infections in part because of higher iron levels.

What to Do If Your Doctor Says You're Iron Deficient or Anemic

Let's consider those cases where women may actually need extra iron to meet their needs. The first case, in which iron supplementation should be approached cautiously, is that of iron-deficiency anemia in menstruating women. You remember Madge, the woman in Chapter 5 who received the diagnosis of anemia from her doctor and went home with some iron supplements. That may be the beginning of a bad habit for Madge, particularly if she continues taking the pills or other tonics later in life. With what we now know about the dangers of excess iron and the exaggeration of the prevalence of anemia, let's take a look at what *you* should do if your doctor says you're anemic.

1. Determine if you really are iron deficient *and* anemic. In Madge's case, the doctor relied on fairly inaccurate estimations for iron deficiency and anemia: the hemoglobin and serum iron tests, both cheap and commonly requested by doctors. If your doctor says you're anemic, ask exactly which tests indicated this. If your doctor used either or both of these screening tests, politely ask for a more detailed analysis, including two or three of the following:

- Serum ferritin test. A result of less than 12 units is considered abnormal.
- Transferrin saturation test. This is equivalent to serum iron divided by TIBC, the total iron-binding capacity; a result of less than 16 percent is considered abnormal.
- Red cell (erythrocyte) protoporphyrin test. A result of *greater* than 70 units, expressed as micrograms per deciliter of red blood cells, is considered abnormal.[3]

If none or only one of these three tests is abnormal, then you can simply stop right there. You could ask that your iron levels be monitored every three to six months, but you do not need to take iron supplements. If your doctor insists on supplementation, get a second opinion.

If, on the other hand, two or three of the test results are abnormal, then indeed you do have iron-deficiency anemia. You should go on to the next step.

2. Determine the cause of your iron-deficiency anemia. Challenge your doctor to determine why you are anemic. Do you have a bad diet or excessive menstrual flow? Do you have anemia as the result of another disease, particularly one that causes blood loss? Have the doctor test for hidden blood in a stool sample; this can indicate whether or not there is bleeding from an ulcer or colon cancer, which often causes anemia. Clearly, a full checkup is in order.

3. Approach iron supplementation cautiously. Dr. William Crosby, the noted iron expert and director of hematology at the

Chapman Cancer Center in Joplin, Missouri, has stated that doctors often prescribe too much iron for their anemic patients.[4,5] In correcting the anemia, the body can only use an extra five or ten milligrams a day, and more than this can be absorbed from a single standard tablet containing 60 milligrams of iron. Still, it is common for doctors to recommend three or four tablets per day. This high dose often leads to more side effects, including heartburn, nausea, upper gastric discomfort, constipation, and diarrhea. Stick to one tablet a day, preferably taken between meals, for no more than one month. Then request the same three tests from your doctor and see if you are okay.

Iron Balance in Pregnancy

The only category of women for which iron supplementation is more than occasionally justified is pregnant women. The demands for iron in pregnancy are quite severe, with 300 milligrams required for the growth of the fetus and 500 milligrams for the expanded blood supply. Most of this extra 800 milligrams of iron is required in the second half of pregnancy.

The large amount of iron required exceeds most women's iron stores. But before getting too concerned, you must realize that nature has endowed the fetus with an extremely effective iron-scavenging ability. Thus, it is not the iron status of the baby that is at stake, but that of the mother.

Without the use of iron supplements, women can often become anemic in the second half of pregnancy. However, the degree of anemia is usually not severe. One factor at work is an enhanced ability of the intestines to absorb iron during pregnancy. And, after birth, the expanded blood supply shrinks back to its normal size, and a great deal of iron is recovered.

The medical community does not have too much confidence in these two positive factors. For some time now iron supplements have been recommended for all pregnant women. The most recent recommendation of the RDA Committee is 30 milligrams of iron per day as a supplement, in addition to 15 milligrams from the diet. The committee recommends that this supplementation should be continued for two to three months after birth to replenish iron stores.[6]

Larger amounts of iron are commonly prescribed without detailed blood analyses of a woman's iron status. Most of the pregnant women I have talked to recently were taking 65 milligrams of iron per day as part of a multivitamin-mineral supplement. Most experts caution that this large amount of iron is only required if the woman is large, has twin fetuses, is in the later stages of pregnancy and has not been taking iron, or is already anemic.

Doctors continue to prescribe too much iron for pregnant women despite a change in the tide among iron experts. High iron intake can needlessly build up a woman's iron stores, especially after birth. One major criticism of this practice is that iron supplementation is not required in the first half of pregnancy because the demands are quite low. One well-regarded obstetrics textbook, *Williams Obstetrics*, recommends that iron supplementation should only be implemented after the first four months of pregnancy.[7] In addition to keeping iron stores from building up, this delay in supplementation will also avoid the risk of aggravating nausea and vomiting, which women often face during the initial months of pregnancy.

Other experts favor the tailoring of iron supplementation to a mother's needs.[8,9] One recent study in Finland revealed that routine iron supplementation is associated with prolonged pregnancy, possibly leading to a number of serious problems for both the fetus and its mother.[10] It is thought that iron supplementation can inhibit intestinal absorption of zinc, which is important in initiating labor. In this study, the group of women who received iron supplements only if they needed them fared much better than those who were supplemented automatically.

The serum ferritin test, which is rarely performed, would be an excellent way to find out if a woman's iron stores are sufficient to carry her through pregnancy. Doctors rely on far too inaccurate means—for example, hemoglobin level and red blood cell concentration—to determine iron status. Ideally, one would like to have a serum ferritin reading of the iron stores at the beginning and the middle of pregnancy. If iron stores are low at any point, then one could begin supplementation. Other indications that a pregnant woman may need iron supplements include a previous bout with iron-deficiency anemia (confirmed by two or more blood tests), dietary inadequacy (for example, from poverty or too much dieting), and chronic blood loss.

Here are the Iron Balance recommendations for pregnant women:

• Insist on a serum ferritin measurement of storage iron at your first checkup. If the serum ferritin reading is less than 10 units, corresponding to fairly low iron stores of less than 100 milligrams, then you are at risk of becoming iron deficient during pregnancy and should begin taking iron supplements immediately.

If the serum ferritin reading is between 10 and 80 units, corresponding to fairly normal iron stores of 100–800 milligrams, then refrain from taking any iron-containing supplement during the first half of pregnancy. To meet the increased needs of other important nutrients, you can take an over-the-counter multivitamin supplement without iron, rather than one of the standard prenatal products. Request an additional serum ferritin test four or five months into your pregnancy. If the reading at that time is less than 10 units, begin iron supplementation.

If the serum ferritin reading is greater than 80 units, corresponding to high iron stores of greater than 800 milligrams, then it is very unlikely that you will become anemic during your pregnancy. Refrain from taking any iron-containing supplement.

• If your doctor says you are severely anemic, if you are carrying twins, or if you are greatly overweight, follow your doctor's recommendations for iron supplementation. However, if you are normal and healthy, I recommend that you ask your doctor to help you find a multivitamin-mineral supplement that contains roughly 30 milligrams of iron per tablet, rather than the 60–65 milligrams that is often present in standard prenatal formulas. You would also save some money by staying away from the prenatal products. For example, prenatal supplements often sell for seventeen to twenty dollars per 100 tablets (Boston area). By comparison, One-A-Day Within Women's Formula (Miles, Inc.) contains plenty of iron (27 milligrams) as well as the folic acid needed in pregnancy (400 micrograms) at a cost of only $6.87 per 100 tablets. (You can even find cheaper generic versions of these supplements with identical compositions; I found one that was $2.00 less than the One-A-Day product.)

• Stop iron supplementation after the birth of your child. As the expanded blood supply collapses, your iron stores are at least partially replaced, and iron supplementation is not needed unless you are clinically anemic. If you are concerned about getting enough nutrients for nursing your child, take a standard multivitamin supplement without iron.

Iron Balance for Infants

After receiving all the iron it needs from the mother to ensure its growth, an infant is born with rather high iron levels. The iron levels are so high that some experts believe that they may be dangerous under certain circumstances. This is especially true for premature infants, particularly those fed high-iron formula or those that require blood transfusions. Though more work needs to be done to understand the effects of iron in premature infants, some scientists believe that certain disorders of prematurity, including those affecting the lungs and eyes, may involve excess iron.[11,12]

The RDA Committee has stated that over the first three months of life a baby does not need any extra iron beyond that present in mother's milk or low-iron formula. The iron content in these foods is 1.5–1.8 milligrams of iron per liter, or .13–.16 milligram per 100 kilocalories.[6]

Despite these recommendations, pediatricians routinely recommend high-iron formula. One recent survey in the state of Washington found that 67 percent of pediatricians never or almost never recommend low-iron formulas with an iron content similar to that of breast milk. Seventeen percent of the physicians interviewed occasionally recommended the low-iron formula for medical reasons or because of parental pressure. Only 16 percent of those interviewed routinely recommended the low-iron formula.[13]

The prevailing approach among pediatricians is clearly to prevent iron-deficiency anemia at all costs. Indeed, they have been extremely successful in fighting this public health problem. Nutritional programs, particularly for the poor, have significantly reduced the incidence of anemia in infants and children over the past thirty years.

Today, however, iron experts, even those who have supported supplementation in the past, are beginning to question the use of high-iron formula. Dr. Peter R. Dallman, an iron expert and pediatrician at the University of California at San Francisco, has recently summarized the debate in the *Journal of Nutrition*.[14] The most likely risk from high-iron formula, he says, is increasing the chance of infection. Bacteria and other organisms can thrive in high-iron environments, particularly in the intestines. Studies have shown conclusively that stool samples from infants fed high-iron formula had a greater number of dangerous bacteria than samples from those fed low-iron formula or breast milk. While it is clear that more research needs to be done to understand the effects of iron on infants and to see if low-iron formula is sufficient to prevent iron deficiency, there appears to be less and less support for going against the RDA Committee recommendations to stick with mother's milk or low-iron formula during the first three months of life.

Iron Balance for Children and Adolescents

When an infant reaches three months of age, the iron levels decrease to more normal values. The requirements for iron then increase as the child develops mentally and physically. From three to six months of age, the RDA Committee recommends a daily intake of 6.6 milligrams of iron. This increases to 8.8 milligrams for infants aged six months to one year, and 10 milligrams for children aged one to ten years. Female adolescents aged ten to eighteen years require 15 milligrams of iron daily, whereas males in that age group need only 12 milligrams.

The incidence of iron deficiency during these crucial years of development must be prevented. Though further research is needed, studies to date have shown that iron-deficient children score significantly lower on both mental and physical tests. They also appear to have shorter attention spans and to be fearful, tired, or tense. A particularly worrisome outcome of some of these studies is that in some cases the deleterious effects of iron deficiency are not corrected after the deficiency has been relieved through supplementation.

The iron requirements for proper mental and physical growth can be obtained with a balanced diet, preferably containing at least some meat. Children raised on vegetarian diets have been shown to be at greater risk for iron deficiency.[15] If a suitable diet is not available, for example in impoverished families, iron supplementation is warranted. The striking drop in the incidence of iron deficiency amongst U.S. children in the past thirty years is due in part to the food assistance, nutritional counseling, and health screening provided by public health efforts like the Women, Infants and Children Program.

The goal in the growth years is to provide sufficient iron for development and to build up a safe level of storage iron, preferably 100–400 milligrams. Periodic blood-iron analyses, including serum ferritin and transferrin saturation measurements, from age one to eighteen will go a long way to ensure that iron deficiency is not present, that iron stores are being established, and that the child does not have hereditary hemochromatosis. When the child reaches eighteen years of age, the effects of too much iron, rather than too little, become most important.

16

Optimal Health Through Optimal Nutrition: The Low-Fat, Low-Iron Life-style

America's table is, slowly but surely, becoming leaner. In the 1970s and 1980s, we witnessed some encouraging changes in the American diet. Beef consumption declined for the first time in the history of the country. The consumption of leaner chicken and fish rose. The word *fiber* entered everyday parlance, as did *cholesterol* and *oat bran*. Despite a confused chorus of experts recommending different strategies, a lot of Americans still got the message: eat less fat and more fruits, vegetables, whole grains, and fiber.

Along the way, a few faint voices from the legions of scientists pointed out that this type of diet could be beneficial not only because it is low in fat but also because it is low in iron. To meet the American Heart Association recommendations of less than 300 milligrams of cholesterol per day and less than 30 percent of calories from fat, one should eat less iron-rich meat. Following the American Cancer Society recommendation to eat more vegetables and high-fiber foods would also lead to reduced iron absorption. Scientists familiar with iron's darker side wondered, "Are low iron levels partly responsible for the preventive effects of these healthy diets?"

But iron's reputation in the medical community was too solid.

180

As the huge anticholesterol machine, the National Cholesterol Education Program, rolled into action in 1985, these questions were barely heard.

We are still at an early stage in defining the proper levels of different nutrients. As we learn more about each of them, we will decrease the recommended amounts of some, increase those amounts for others, and perhaps even add some new ones. This whole process takes time. Getting scientists, physicians, and nutritionists to agree on something is quite a feat. In the case of iron, a great deal of the scientific information has yet to filter up to those individuals who make policy and issue recommendations.

The idea that low iron levels would be healthiest fits in well with recent trends in nutrition. We have moved away from the idea that megadoses of vitamin C or E can save us, and, for the potentially dangerous nutrients, we seem to be moving in the direction of "less is best." For example, the "safe" range for cholesterol levels seems to be decreasing all the time. The latest findings from a study conducted by Dr. Dean Ornish, assistant clinical professor of medicine at the University of California at San Francisco and president of the Preventive Medicine Institute in nearby Sausalito, show that heart disease patients can actually unclog their arteries, but only if they stick to an extremely low-fat, vegetarian diet and lower their cholesterol levels drastically. Patients in this study who followed the less stringent American Heart Association dietary recommendations failed to improve.[1]

In looking forward to designing the optimal diet for *Homo sapiens* (that's us), it pays to look back in time as well. When we do so, we see that our ancestors were fairly strict practitioners of the low-fat–low-iron life-style.

Back to the Jungle

The human body was designed for what type of diet? Scientists believe that we evolved on a diet not unlike that of the chimpanzee and other primates with whom we share common ancestors. While early humans ate meat when they could get it, it was largely vegetables and fruits that sustained them.

Though not easy to obtain, there is archeological evidence supporting our vegetarian heritage. The collections of animal bones and hunting tools found in the remains of early camps exaggerate the importance of meat over plant food which, by comparison, left few remains. An analysis of our teeth and jaws reveals that they are most suitable for grinding plant food; we lack the sharp, meat-tearing teeth of carnivorous animals like dogs. In addition, our long digestive tracts seem better designed for the slow processing of plant food. This is in contrast to the shorter digestive pathways in carnivores.[2]

A clearer glimpse of our dietary origins comes from studies of isolated modern-day tribes, most of whom have never seen a car or a modern building. These tribes of Africa and South America are often referred to as hunter-gatherers. The men often attempt to hunt during the day while the women collect plant foods around their camp. With only primitive hunting tools, the hunt is often not successful, and the men come home empty-handed. It is up to the women to gather enough food from the lush surroundings to sustain them. *Gatherer-hunters* would perhaps be a more fitting characterization of these people.[3,4]

Let's take a closer look at the striking contrast between this diet and our own.

Kumsa is a forty-year-old !Kung bushman living in southern Africa. (The exclamation point represents one of the many clicking sounds used in the !Kung language.) These people, also known as the San, are among the best-studied modern tribes. Kumsa often goes out hunting with the other men from his village, marching five to fifteen miles for up to ten hours a day, three days a week. More often than not, the hunters return home with little or nothing to cook on the spit. Meanwhile, Kumsa's wife //Kushe (the // symbol represents the clicking sound one would use to urge on a horse) and the other women of the village have spent an average of one to three hours picking fruits and vegetables from trees and bushes and digging for tubers and special roots. Twenty-three plants make up 90 percent of the !Kung diet. One of these is the mongongo nut; its edible fruit and kernel together are as nutritious as peanuts or soybeans. Another popular item is the baobab fruit, a delectable treat high in vitamin C. The tsien bean is also a mainstay of the !Kung diet, as are various berries, tubers, roots and melons.[5]

In contrast, Tom, your average American, has no problem getting as much meat as he wants. He may eat one serving of meat in his sandwich at lunch and probably the equivalent of two servings at dinner. The domestic meat he consumes is derived from grain-fed, grazing livestock and is higher in saturated fat than the flesh of any lean, wild animals which Kumsa might be fortunate enough to kill. The rest of Tom's diet does little to make up for this bad start. Even if he has begun eating a high-fiber cereal for breakfast, it is doubtful that he gets enough fiber, fruit, and vegetables at each meal. Too much of his protein and calories come from meat.

We can look at two biochemical parameters and easily distinguish the healthier of the two men.

	Serum Cholesterol *(milligrams per deciliter)*
Kumsa	120
Tom	225

	Total Amount of Stored Iron *(milligrams)*
Kumsa	400
Tom	1400

That the hunter-gatherer vegetarian diet leads to lower cholesterol levels is widely known. This is surely a major factor why societies that subsist on this type of diet are free from many of the chronic diseases of affluence, such as heart disease, cancer, stroke, diabetes, osteoporosis, and high blood pressure. The large difference in iron levels, on the other hand, has been overlooked, but this surely contributes to the relative health and vitality of the more primitive peoples.

"We're Basically a Vegetarian Species"

Throughout human history, great societies have subsisted on largely vegetarian diets. The Chinese and Japanese diets are based on rice; the Babylonians, Egyptians, Romans, and Greeks ate wheat; and the Mayas, Incas, and Aztecs of the Americas ate corn and beans. Where old-fashioned diets are still consumed, people are clearly healthier in many ways. A recent study of 6,500 people in China, where heart disease and colon cancer rates are fractions of those in the U.S., provides a good example.[6] With only 7 percent of their protein on average coming from animal products, their cholesterol and iron levels are close to those of the !Kung bush people. The average blood cholesterol level is around 130 milligrams per 100 milliliters, and the total iron stores in men are around 700 milligrams, both far lower than those for most Americans and people in other Western countries.

Our growing understanding of the potential health risks of high iron levels has coincided with calls for a more vegetarian life-style for those of us in Western countries. Study after study has shown that vegetarians are healthier. A recent position paper of the American Dietetic Association underlined these facts:[7]

> . . . a considerable body of scientific data suggests positive relationships between a vegetarian lifestyle and risk reduction for several chronic degenerative diseases and conditions, such as obesity, coronary artery disease, hypertension, diabetes mellitus, colon cancer, and others. . . . Vegetarians also have lower rates of osteoporosis, lung and breast cancer, kidney stones, gallstones, and diverticular disease.
>
> It is the position of the ADA that vegetarian diets are healthful and nutritionally adequate when appropriately planned.

From what we know about our dietary heritage, it appears that Homo sapiens is best designed for a diet of fruits, vegetables, and grains rather than one that is high in meat. Dr. T. Colin Campbell, a nutritional biochemist at Cornell University and the director of the large Chinese study mentioned previously, has stated, "We're basically a vegetarian species and should be eating a wide variety of plant foods and minimizing our intake of animal foods."[6] One physicians' group, the Physicians Committee for Responsible Medicine, has even advocated the replacement of the four basic food groups—originally fruits and vegetables, grain, dairy products, and meats—with a new "basic four": fruits, grains, vegetables, and legumes, such as beans, peanut butter, and soybeans. The committee recommended that meats and dairy products should play a lesser role in the American diet.[8]

Meat: A Trojan Horse for Iron

Excessive meat intake has been indicted as a major contributing factor behind many of the chronic illnesses that plague Western countries. A lot of attention has been focused on how excessive meat consumption raises the intake of saturated fat and cholesterol and displaces healthier fare such as fruits, vegetables, and grains. These links are now well established, and they alone should convince you to curb your desire for too many juicy steaks.

But there is more to the story.

You see, every bite of meat can raise not only your cholesterol level but also your iron level. Meat contains a powerful one-two punch of saturated fats and cholesterol on the one hand and easily absorbable iron on the other. Iron in meat, unlike the iron in other foods, is chemically attached to a sort of Trojan Horse (known as *heme*) that sneaks it into your intestinal cells with relative ease. And, unfortunately, our bodies do not seem to have a way to decrease the percentage of meat iron absorbed from the diet when our iron stores are sufficient. While the absorption of plant-based iron will decrease in high-iron folks, meat iron just keeps on coming.[9]

Though there are many contributing factors to one's iron level, it is well known that people who eat less meat over a significant period of time have lower iron levels. Several studies have shown, for example, that vegetarians have lower iron stores than the rest of the omnivorous population. And people in countries with high per-capita meat intake generally have higher iron levels. Australians, who invite us to come "down under" and share a slab of meat cooked up "on the barbie"—the barbecue—have one of the highest per-capita meat intakes in the world. A recent survey of almost 2000 employees in a large bank and an insurance company in Australia shows that their iron levels are indeed very high, with men having around 2000 milligrams of storage iron.[10] The meat intake and iron levels of Americans are comparable to that of Australians. As mentioned above, the Chinese and other Asians as well eat less meat and have much lower iron levels. People in countries such as Sweden and Finland seem to lie in between these extremes.

The Vegetarian Route to Lower Iron Levels

Why is the vegetarian diet low on iron? The iron in fruits, vegetables and grains is not bound to any Trojan Horse that helps it enter the intestinal cells. It must fend for itself, as it tries to disentangle itself from food and then penetrate the intestines. Only about 2 to 10 percent of this form of iron is absorbed from the diet, and this amount decreases as the iron stores in the body are established. While vitamin C and other food constituents can increase the amount of iron absorption, the iron uptake in vegetarians is still less than that of omnivores.

Phytic Acid, a Sponge for Excess Iron

One of the major factors reponsible for the low absorption of iron from plant-based foods is phytic acid, a phosphorus-rich substance that is particularly abundant in whole grains and certain nuts and legumes. Phytic acid grabs on to the iron in food and reduces the amount of iron available for uptake by the intestinal cells.

The effects of phytic acid on iron absorption have been known for years. Studies dating back to the 1940s show that subjects eating phytic acid–rich whole-grain breads absorb *less* iron than those eating white bread, even though the whole-grain bread has 50 percent *more* iron.[11] The milling process that removes so many good nutrients and fiber also removes phytic acid: white bread has five to twenty times less phytic acid than whole-grain bread. It is no wonder that people in Western countries have such high iron levels: we strip our bread of this protective substance, and then we fortify it with *extra* iron!

As mentioned in Chapter 11, Dr. Ernst Graf of the Pillsbury Company and Dr. John Eaton, a professor at the University of Minnesota in Minneapolis, proposed in 1985 that phytic acid could be an important substance that naturally protects us from colon cancer.[12] They showed that phytic acid surrounds iron in the intestines in such a way as to prevent the metal from assisting in the production of dangerous, cancer-causing chemicals.[13] In addition, lower amounts of available iron would reduce the growth rate of small tumors which desperately need iron to divide and conquer.

The proposal of Drs. Graf and Eaton—that phytic acid is a sponge for excess iron in our colon—is supported by large population studies that found that people who eat a lot of whole-grain products are less likely to die from colon cancer. The usual explanation for these results is that it is the high fiber content in the diet that is protective. Fiber, the nondigestible portion of food, is thought to dilute the harmful carcinogens present in the bowel and hasten bowel movements. But if fiber is responsible, then why do the studies fail to show any correlation between the consumption of high-fiber fruits and vegetables and protection from colon cancer?[14,15] It is only the whole-grain cereals that seem to work, and *these are precisely the foods that are richest in phytic acid*.

Differences in phytic-acid consumption among the people of Finland and Denmark may explain why the Finns have lower colon cancer rates than the culturally and ethnically similar Danes.[12] Both societies eat too much high-fat foods, particularly from dairy products, and suffer from high rates of heart disease. The high fat intake is also thought to promote colon cancer. However, the Finns have somehow escaped this curse; they have a third to half the colon cancer rate in Denmark.

The key reason is thought to be the large quantities of unrefined grain products in the Finnish diet, particularly rye and whole wheat. In contrast, the Danes are somewhat more fond of pastries—hence, the "Danish"—and other foods made from refined wheat flour. Clearly, the Finns consume more phytic acid. In the next chapter, you will learn a few tips from the Finns on how to increase your intake of this "sponge for iron."

Swimming Upstream: Living the Low-Fat, Low-Iron Life-style Today

Though it looks like it is going to take some time, Americans do appear to be changing their dietary habits for the better. The consumption of beef and pork has begun to decline as people have begun to eat more cereal, pasta, and fish. It is not clear whether these improvements are linked to the decreased mortality rate from heart disease, which has been declining for thirty years, but they nevertheless are a step in the right direction.

Other broader issues may push many people toward the vegetarian life-style. As people become more sensitized to environmental and hunger issues, the words of Frances Moore Lappé, author of *Diet for a Small Planet*, and others may be heeded. As Lappé pointed out, our farms are losing topsoil because we are growing so much grain and soy to feed our cows; some sixteen pounds of feed ends up yielding only one pound of beef.[16] Why not eat the cereals ourselves? They are much healthier fare anyway.

From a hunger standpoint, the statistics are astounding. Livestock ate a third of the world's grain output in 1970; today the amount is half. Just think of how many more mouths could be fed if we reduced our consumption of meat.

Animal rights issues, too, have nudged many people toward the vegetarian way of life. Several public action groups have gained strength in recent years. While some of these are unfairly critical of the need for animals in health research, others responsibly focus on minimizing the pain that animals experience and convincing the public of the virtues of the vegetarian way of life.

Nonetheless, if you take a close, hard look at what America is eating, most people still fall far short of the recommendations of the American Heart Association and the American Cancer Society.

What is standing in our way? Well, for one thing, we love meat. We love the taste of it and its texture. Along with our ancestral cousin, the monkey, we humans have always eaten as much meat as we could get our hands on. Our brains are big, but not big enough to tell us when to stop. Meat has become a health threat only in relatively recent times, in which farming provides bountiful quantities of fatty meat and refrigeration has prolonged its shelf life.

There are also important social factors that keep us chewing on the flesh. For one, meat is a status symbol. In the days of the hunter-gatherers, men would get a great deal of prestige from obtaining meat. For some people, meat also has a connotation of masculinity and power. Frances Lappé once heard of a man who refused to become a vegetarian because he believed he would not be able to make love to his wife afterward!

Meat is also a centerpiece for socialization in our culture. From the earliest days of humankind onward, a family or tribe would gather around a kill while a man performed a carving ceremony. This tradition continues today in many homes during Thanksgiving and Christmas holidays.

Vegetarians are up against a lot in this world, especially when they try to get others to join their cause. The uphill battle can be seen in the following excerpt from an Associated Press article from March 1990 entitled "National Meatless Day Attracts Only Scant Support":[17]

> Not everyone noticed, but the sixth annual Great American Meatout was held yesterday, a one-day boycott of meat sponsored by the Farm Animal Reform Movement, a national advocacy group opposed to "factory farming" and in favor of vegetarian diets.
>
> Among the events held yesterday around the country, soup kitchens went vegetarian in Pittsburgh, students demonstrated at a cheese-steak restaurant in Philadelphia and the Mayor of Des Moines offered his support, to the dismay of some other Iowans.
>
> "You're not my Mayor," was among the kinder remarks

greeting Mayor John (Pat) Dorrian at the Iowa Statehouse after he signed a proclamation recognizing the one-day meat boycott in the capital of the nation's top pork producing state. . . .

[The event had some success in Pittsburgh but not] in Philadelphia, home of the cheese steak, where Meatout supporters gathered at Jim's Steaks on South Street. A group of teen-age vegetarians stood outside the Art Deco landmark passing out anti-meat fliers, carrots and orange slices as the aroma of seared beef and fried onions wafted overhead.

But they were unable to persuade many in the early lunch crowd to avoid meat for a day. . . . "What is this, save a cow?" said Bernie Bartholome, a New York businessman, as he ate a cheese steak laden with peppers, onions and tomatoes. "See, I eat vegetables, too."

Perhaps slowly is the only way label-conscious Americans are going to convert to a healthier diet. One vegetarian doctor recommends this type of diet for his patients, but he warns, "I never use the 'V' word. It scares people away."

Most experts are recommending that people gradually change their diet for the better. Switching to low-fat or nonfat milk, eating leaner cuts of meat, and cutting down on those quick trips to McDonald's are all a good place to start. Pick up a good vegetarian cookbook and try a new recipe. Try using meat as a side dish rather than the centerpiece of the meal.

As you will see in the following chapter, many of the steps you should be taking to minimize fat intake will also reduce your iron intake. This makes the Iron Balance diet easy. And, if you love meat, don't worry: you'll learn how to get by on tasty low-fat, low-iron selections.

17

The Iron Balance Diet

You can live the low-fat, low-iron life-style by including a few simple dietary practices in the commonsense low-fat approach recommended by the American Cancer Society and the American Heart Association. A low-fat diet is in fact the foundation of the Iron Balance diet; some of the rules are very similar. If you are unfamiliar with the traditional low-fat recommendations, you can refer to a number of excellent books, such as *Jane Brody's Good Food Book* (New York: W.W. Norton & Co., 1985; New York: Bantam, 1987) and *The American Heart Association Low-Fat, Low-Cholesterol Cookbook* by Dr. Scott Grundy and Mary Winston (New York: Times Books, 1989).

What will the Iron Balance diet do for you? First, it will prevent the excessive buildup of iron in amounts above your present level. Second, it may, over time, decrease the iron levels in your body. You need to realize that if you are starting out with fairly high iron levels, as indicated in your self-test score or a serum ferritin measurement performed by your doctor, you will need to take additional measures to reduce your iron levels to the theoretical safe range. The most important of these additional measures, blood donation, is discussed in the next chapter.

Presented in this chapter are the Iron Balance dietary recommendations, many of which are simple but revolutionary and cannot be found in any other health book. These health tips are then put together into a sample menu, which you can adapt and vary to your particular tastes. And finally, for those of you who have tried different weight-loss or low-fat diets in the past, the final section of this chapter will show you how the iron content in these diets compares to that of the Iron Balance diet.

The Iron Balance Dietary Recommendations

Here, in a nutshell, are the four major Iron Balance dietary recommendations:

1. Do not take supplements that contain iron or eat foods that are highly fortified with iron.
2. Eat less meat and more fruits, vegetables, and grains.
3. Eat foods rich in phytic acid, such as wheat bran, rye, and whole wheat products.
4. Keep your alcohol consumption to a minimum.

Depending on your preferences, you may also want to consider these additional tips:

- Try not to eat foods rich in vitamin C (such as citrus fruits) or take vitamin C supplements during meals or within two hours afterward.
- If you like tea or coffee, drink some with your meals or within an hour after you eat.
- Do not cook with iron pots.

Let's go over each one of these recommendations in detail and see how you can easily incorporate them into your diet.

1. Do Not Take Supplements That Contain Iron or Eat Foods That Are Highly Fortified in Iron

Iron supplements should only be taken under doctor's orders. Unless your doctor has diagnosed you as being anemic and requiring iron supplementation, you have no business taking iron pills or even multivitamin-mineral supplements that contain high quantities of iron. The extra iron buildup that you acquire from these products will do you no good and can only do you harm in the long run. Furthermore, even if your doctor *has* diagnosed you as being anemic, please follow the recommendations in Chapter 15 for challenging the diagnosis, finding the cause of the anemia, and making sure that you do not take too much iron in resolving the problem.

This Iron Balance recommendation is probably most relevant in the choice of your morning breakfast cereal. As you know from Chapter 6, the food industry has eagerly embraced the recommendations of the U.S. government for nutrient intake and has packed a whole day's worth of nutrition into a single bowl of cereal. But you do not need 18 milligrams of iron (100 percent of the RDA) to start off your day. Nor do you need 8 milligrams (45 percent of the RDA). Many popular cereals contain this much added iron. I recommend that you try to select cereals with iron contents of 25 percent of the U.S. RDA or less (see table in Chapter 6). I will have more to say about which cereals to select in discussing the third dietary recommendation regarding phytic acid. As you will see, choosing the proper cereal will reduce the absorption of fortified iron, as long as iron is present in no more than moderate amounts.

2. Eat Less Meat and More Fruits, Vegetables, and Grains

This rule is at the heart of the new low-fat, low-iron, high-fiber diet. Replacing meat with low-calorie foods will not only reduce your intake of fat, cholesterol, and iron but it will also help you lose weight.

Now, if you are already a vegetarian or if you only very rarely eat meat, that's great! As long as you eat a variety of protein sources such as grains, legumes, and low-fat dairy products, you will have the healthiest possible diet, one that is probably the closest to the diet for which the human body was designed.

But if you are like me and cannot give up meat, you can still go a long way to ensure that you are not poisoning your body with excess fat, cholesterol, and iron. Here are some tips:

Try to eat meat only once a day. If you can eat pasta or salad at lunch, reward yourself at night with your favorite meat dish.

Eat smaller portions of meat. One serving of meat is generally considered to be three or four ounces, a little more than a regular McDonald's hamburger patty. The American idea of one serving of meat, however, is often a large, juicy, inch-thick steak, which is often equivalent to two to three servings.

Choose lean cuts. With the nation's health consciousness on the rise, these are becoming more available in the grocery store and in "enlightened" restaurants.

Fish and poultry are your best bets for low fat and *low iron.* Take a look at Figure 17-1, a chart ranking meats from the healthiest choices to the worst. As you might have guessed purely on the basis of its low fat content, fish gets the blue ribbon. But fish is also low in iron![1] Nature has made it easy for us to make the right choices: iron and fat, more or less, go hand in hand. (As you may know, many fish, such as salmon, trout, halibut, bluefish, sardines, and bass, are also good choices because they contain substantial quantities of omega-3 fatty acids, substances thought to decrease the clotting action of the blood and possibly prevent heart attacks.)

We should all be trying to eat more fish, fresh or frozen. You needn't worry about the safety of our fish supply: most of the concerns focus on *raw* shellfish, which does cause illness more often than other forms of meat. But the risk of illness from *cooked* fish is only around one illness in five million servings.[2]

Going down the list of meat choices in Figure 17-1, you will see that chicken and turkey take second place. The fat and iron content of these poultry selections is only slightly higher than fish. While many experts feel that it is the low fat content that

RANKING MEATS FOR THE LOW-FAT, LOW-IRON LIFESTYLE

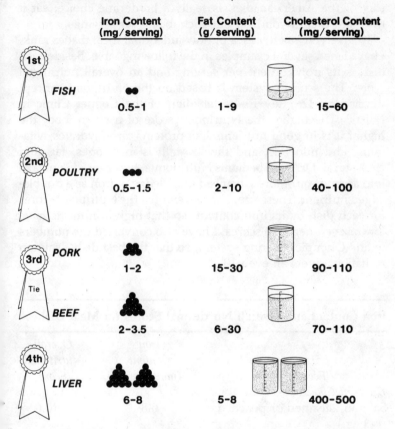

		Iron Content (mg/serving)	Fat Content (g/serving)	Cholesterol Content (mg/serving)
1st	FISH	0.5–1	1–9	15–60
2nd	POULTRY	0.5–1.5	2–10	40–100
3rd	PORK	1–2	15–30	90–110
Tie	BEEF	2–3.5	6–30	70–110
4th	LIVER	6–8	5–8	400–500

Figure 17-1. Ranking meats for the low-fat, low-iron life-style. This chart shows how various meats stack up in terms of both fat-cholesterol and iron content. In general, the higher the fat-cholesterol content, the higher the iron content. The meats we already know to be lower in fat—fish, chicken, and turkey—are also lower in iron.

makes fish and poultry the healthiest choices, we may find out in five or ten years that their low iron content is equally important.

The remaining meat choices—pork, beef, and liver—are less healthy. We can see that liver, in particular, is especially toxic:

it is extremely high in both cholesterol and iron. Beef, the main-stay of the American diet, is really a borderline choice: eat it now and then if you like, but stick to smaller servings.

To give you a better idea of how individual meat dishes rank, I have listed several examples in the following table. Beside each dish is its iron content per serving and an overall nutritional score. The scoring system is based on the Nutripoint concept devised by Dr. Roy E. Vartabedian of the Cooper Clinic in Dallas.[3] The higher the Nutripoint score of a given food, the higher it is in good nutrients like protein, carbohydrates, vitamins, and minerals, and the lower it is in calories, fat, and cholesterol. Dr. Vartabedian's Nutripoints, however, do not take into account our more advanced knowledge of iron as a double-edged nutrient. Therefore, I have weighted the Nutripoint scores for each dish by its iron content, so that high-iron meats have low or even negative scores. I have also converted the numbers to an "Olympic" scoring system, so that the best dish—salmon or halibut—gets an even 10.

Iron Content and Overall Nutritional Scores for Meat Dishes

Food Item	Iron Content (milligrams)	Overall Nutritional Score
Excellent Choices		
Salmon, steamed or poached (3 oz.)	0.8	10.0
Halibut, baked (4 oz.)	0.9	10.0
Swordfish, baked (3 oz.)	1.0	8.0
Tuna, canned in water (¾ cup)	2.3	7.5
Good Choices		
Turkey, light meat, baked, without skin (3 oz.)	1.0	5.0
Chicken breast, baked, without skin (3 oz.)	1.1	4.0
Rabbit, domestic (3 oz.)	1.3	2.0

Food Item	Iron Content (milligrams)	Overall Nutritional Score
Borderline Choices		
Pork chop, loin, lean, baked (3 oz.)	2.2	0.5
Beef, round steak, lean, broiled (3 oz.)	3.2	0.0
Hamburger patty, lean, broiled (3 oz.)	2.6	−0.5
Ham, lean, baked, canned, 4% fat (4 oz.)	4.3	−0.5
Bad Choices		
Bacon, fried (3 pieces)	0.8	−3.0
Beef liver, fried (3 oz.)	7.5	−3.5
Frankfurter, beef (1)	0.8	−5.5
Awful Choice		
Sausage link, pork (2)	1.6	−7.0

Below are two additional tables for people "on the go." As you can see, I did not have much luck finding "excellent" or "good" choices among frozen meat dinners and fast food. I could not even find any with positive scores! The scores are low largely because of the high fat content of these prepared foods. The fat not only comes from the meat but also from the "special sauces." However, the high iron content in many of the fast foods, particularly those with large portions of beef, drags the scores down even further. Clearly, the big loser in these two categories is the McDonald's McDLT hamburger, with an abysmal −17.7 score: it's loaded with fat and cholesterol, along with 6.6 milligrams of iron!

(McDonald's announced in 1991 the development of a new low-fat burger—the McLean Deluxe—with roughly half of the fat of a Quarter Pounder.[4] But don't be fooled. While the sandwich is better for you than the Quarter Pounder, preliminary dietary analyses suggest that it will still rank in the "Bad Choices" category.)

Iron Content and Overall Nutritional Scores for Frozen Meat Dinners

Food Item	Iron Content (milligrams)	Overall Nutritional Score
Excellent and Good Choices		
None		
Borderline Choices		
Turkey breast, sliced with mushroom sauce; Stouffer's	0.7	0.0
Chicken and pasta divan; Healthy Choice	1.8	0.0
Chicken parmigiana; Healthy Choice	2.7	0.0
Beef Oriental pepper steak; Healthy Choice	1.4	−1.0
Turkey breast; Healthy Choice	1.8	−1.0
Beef sirloin tips; Healthy Choice	2.7	−1.0
Chicken imperial; Weight Watchers	1.8	−1.5
Bad Choices		
Beef Oriental with vegetables and rice; Stouffer's	1.4	−3.0
Chicken cacciatore with vermicelli; Stouffer's	2.7	−4.5

Food Item	Iron Content (milligrams)	Overall Nutritional Score
Awful Choices		
Turkey breast, stuffed; Weight Watchers	1.8	−7.0
Beef Salisbury steak with Italian Sauce; Stouffer's	2.7	−7.0

Iron Content and Overall Nutritional Scores for Fast Food

Food Item	Iron Content (milligrams)	Overall Nutritional Score
Excellent, Good, and Borderline Choices None		
Bad Choices		
Taco Bell beef taco (1)	1.2	−4.0
Burger King hamburger (1)	2.7	−4.0
McDonald's hamburger (1)	2.9	−4.0
McDonald's Chicken McNuggets (1 serving)	1.3	−4.5
Burger King ham and cheese sandwich (1)	3.2	−4.5
Roast beef sandwich (1)	4.0	−4.5
Awful Choices		
Burger King Whaler sandwich (1)	2.2	−6.0
Kentucky Fried Chicken, drumsticks (2 pieces)	1.2	−7.0
Kentucky Fried Chicken, wings (2 pieces)	0.9	−7.5
Kentucky Fried Chicken, breasts (2 pieces)	1.6	−7.5

Food Item	Iron Content (milligrams)	Overall Nutritional Score
McDonald's Filet-O-Fish (1)	2.5	−7.5
Burger King chicken sandwich (1)	3.3	−7.5
McDonald's Quarter Pounder (1)	4.3	−10.0
Burger King bacon double cheeseburger (1)	3.8	−11.0
Kentucky Fried Chicken, thighs (2 pieces)	2.1	−12.0
McDonald's Big Mac (1)	4.9	−12.5
Burger King Whopper sandwich with cheese (1)	4.9	−12.5
McDonald's McDLT (1)	6.6	−17.7

3. Eat Foods Rich in Phytic Acid, Such as Wheat Bran, Rye, and Whole Wheat Products

Phytic acid, also known as *phytate*, is the substance in whole grains, legumes, and nuts that acts as a sponge for excess iron in your intestines. By eating phytate-rich foods at most of your meals, you can protect your colon from iron-catalyzed chemical reactions and minimize the amount of iron you absorb from plant-based foods.[5,6]

The first of these two effects of phytate is also thought to protect seeds from decomposition. Despite high concentrations of fat and iron, a chemically reactive combination when in the presence of oxygen, seeds can remain viable for up to four hundred years. It is thought that the high phytate content of seeds keeps the iron in its place and prevents it from starting any trouble.[6]

As discussed in the previous chapter, the Finns stand out as heavy phytate consumers. This may be an important reason why they have very low colon cancer rates. What is the Finnish secret? If you look at food consumption charts issued by the Organization for Economic Cooperation and Development, the most notable feature of the Finnish diet is a very high consumption of rye, the grain with the highest overall phytate content.[7] From 1976 to 1985, for example, Finland ranked first in per-capita rye consumption, with fifty or sixty grams per person per day, equivalent to around three slices of rye bread a day. The people in rural areas eat more rye than city dwellers, and this may be one reason why the country folk have lower colon-cancer mortality rates.[8]

Rye is important to Finland and other northern European countries because it can grow where it is too cold for other grains. The Finns eat it morning, noon, and night. Instead of oatmeal for breakfast, many eat *ruispuuro*, literally "rye porridge," a hearty start for a cold, dark winter day. Their rye bread, *ruisleipä*, which accompanies every meal in large quantities, is a dark sourdough version; that of Sweden, on the other hand, is sweeter. Dry, flat rye crackers (*näkkileipä* in Finnish, *knäckerbröd* in Swedish) are also popular in Scandinavia. A unique Finnish invention containing rye is a funny sort of fish sandwich, *kalakukko*, in which fish is wrapped in bacon and baked inside rye bread.[9]

You can get some rye into your diet by simply eating rye bread. Or you can try those Swedish flatbread crackers made from rye. They are available in most grocery stores, and with *no* fat and few calories, they are great if you are trying to lose some weight.

To get some variety into your phytate choices, select your favorite foods from the table below. Between whole grains and certain legumes, you can always ensure ample phytate at each meal. If you eat phytate-rich wheat bran at breakfast, you can even beat the Finns in total phytate intake. Try to find whole-bran cereals without added iron (such as Nabisco's 100% Bran) in your grocery or health-food store.

Here's a rule of thumb to keep in mind when you are looking for phytate-rich breads: the heavier, the better. The yeast used to raise dough and make it lighter has special enzymes that decompose the valuable phytate. The longer the dough is allowed to rise, the more time the enzyme has to destroy the phytate. Rising times of two hours or more can lead to the loss of 10 to 50 percent or more of the original phytate content.[10]

Phytate-Rich Foods for Different Meals

	Phytic Acid Content[5,6,10,11] (percentage of dry weight)
BREAKFAST	
Excellent choices	
Wheat bran cereals like All-Bran	3.0–5.0%
Oatmeal	2.4%
Raisin bran	1.8%
Good choices	
Shredded wheat	1.5%
Rye bread	0.8–1.5%
Whole wheat bread	0.6–1.0%
Special K	0.7%
Product 19	0.5%
Poor choices	
Rice Krispies	0.24%
Pumpernickel bread	0.16%
White bread or French bread	0.03–0.13%
Cornflakes	0.05%
Raisin bread	0.09%
LUNCH AND DINNER	
Excellent choices	
Lima beans	0.9–2.5%
Wild rice	2.2%
Red kidney beans	1.2–2.1%
Pinto beans	0.6–2.0%
Navy beans	1.8%

	Phytic Acid Content[5,6,10,11] (percentage of dry weight)
Good choices	
Rye bread	0.8–1.5%
Corn bread	1.4%
Soybeans	1.4%
Peas	0.9–1.2%
Whole wheat bread	0.6–1.0%
Barley	1.0%
Brown rice	0.9%
Corn	0.9%

SNACKS OR CONDIMENTS (SEEDS AND NUTS)

Excellent choices

Sesame seeds	5.3%
Pumpkin seeds	4.3%
Sunflower seeds	1.9%
Peanuts	1.9%

4. Keep Your Alcohol Consumption to a Minimum

You might think it odd that this time-honored proscription is one of the major Iron Balance dietary recommendations. What does alcohol have to do with iron? Plenty. The more we learn, the more it looks like the damaging effects of alcohol and iron go hand in hand.

A number of studies have shown that heavy drinkers, even those without irreversible damage to their livers, have high iron levels.[12,13] The same holds true for adolescents who either drink occasionally or more often.[14] It has also been found that iron levels can return to normal if these individuals stop drinking alcohol altogether.

There are a variety of reasons why alcohol might increase iron levels, though doctors are not sure which are most important. Alcohol increases the acidity of the digestive tract, and this in turn is thought to increase the absorption of iron from all foods except meat. Alcohol also slows down the manufacture of iron-rich red blood cells, freeing up a good deal of iron, which is simply added to existing stores. In addition, it appears that alcohol-induced tissue damage, particularly in the liver, disrupts the ability of a cell to prevent iron from entering.

Recent animal studies by researchers in France and the United States indicate that this disruption in the normal cellular protocol for handling iron may be at the root of alcohol's evil ways.[15-17] Liver and brain samples from drunk rats show an alarming increase in the amount of "bad" iron—the unrestrained, mischievous kind—inside cells. Alcohol is like an evil spirit that enlists unwitting iron atoms to join the dark forces. This form of iron creates the bad chemistry that appears to lead to two of the most devastating effects of alcohol abuse, liver cirrhosis and brain damage.

The research in this area has not progressed to the point that we know whether or not lower iron levels might protect us from some of the adverse effects of alcohol. But we do know that liver damage in people with very high iron levels due to inherited iron-overload disease is exacerbated by drinking. The best advice for now is obvious: to be on the safe side, you should minimize the levels of both iron *and* alcohol in your body.

How much alcohol can you drink and still be healthy? In the 1990 dietary guidelines released by the U.S. government, men are advised to have no more than two drinks a day.[18] Since women break down alcohol more slowly, they are advised to have no more than one drink a day. (One drink is defined as 12 ounces of ordinary beer, 5 ounces of wine, or 1.5 ounces of distilled spirits.)

This advice has been around for a long time. Most conventional experts believe that one or two drinks a day causes no adverse effects in otherwise healthy individuals. Furthermore, moderate drinking is thought to decrease the risk of heart disease by slightly increasing the amount of protective, "good" cholesterol in the blood. These beliefs, coupled with mankind's love of alcohol and the powerful liquor industry, have ingrained in us the notion that this one toxic substance is somehow special: it seems to be okay for everyday use.

I think we ought to slip off the party hats and take a close, hard look at the facts. First, we still do not know enough about the potential for subtle, gradual damage that alcohol may cause. A toxin is a toxin, even if it is socially popular. As people live longer, the chronic effects of alcohol may be disguised as other diseases, or they may be accepted as simply the effects of old age. Second, the finding that drinking adjusts our blood chemistry a little—which gave many people a good excuse to drink—is scientifically interesting but hardly a basis for public health policy. And the logic of adding one toxin, alcohol, to help us deal with another, cholesterol, escapes me.

For these reasons, I can only recommend that you stop drinking altogether or at least limit yourself to perhaps one to three drinks *per week*. Here are some suggestions:

Cut down on your total alcohol intake by drinking only on social occasions; for example, on weekends. A couple of drinks on the weekend is better than fourteen drinks during the week.

When you do drink, do so only when you are in a good mood, not stressed out or depressed. Use some activity other than drinking—exercise, a hobby, a good book or movie—to relax. You may find that when you are in a good mood, you may end up not drinking at all, and if you do drink, you will drink less.

On your nondrinking days, try a nonalcoholic beer or wine. Nonalcoholic beer is becoming more popular as people become more health conscious. Companies have improved upon the brewing process, and some of the selections are not bad. If you are willing to try a number of them, I am sure you will find one that is full-bodied and thirst-quenching.

Minor Tips

If you follow the four major Iron Balance dietary recommendations, you will have come a long way in correcting your natural high-iron habits. There are also some minor tips that, if they are not nearly as important as those already discussed, are well worth knowing. These are things that depend a great deal on personal preference and will have only moderate effects on your total body iron load. Keep them in the back of your mind when you are in the kitchen.

Try Not to Eat Foods Rich in Vitamin C (Such As Citrus Fruits) or Take Vitamin C Supplements During or Within Two Hours After Meals

If you have ever taken vitamin C to help you get over a cold, you have joined millions of people, including myself, who became "sold on C" as a cure for anything from colds to cancer. Passionate and well-meaning scientists, armed with excellent ideas and the results from innumerable test-tube and animal studies, continue to push for higher RDAs for this most celebrated of vitamins. Vitamin C is absolutely required for the proper synthesis of collagen, the glue that holds our tissues together. It also has many other important functions, such as assisting in the production of chemicals in the brain that transmit signals from one cell to another. However, large clinical studies have failed to provide proof that vitamin C prevents colds or helps people get over them faster. And most experts feel that evidence linking vitamin C to cancer prevention is a little weak. In addition, they worry that large doses can cause serious side effects, such as kidney stones and excessive iron absorption.[19]

The enhancement of iron absorption caused by vitamin C has led many to believe that this was an important role for the vitamin in the early days when humans were not the walking rust pots they are today. Vitamin C greases the wheels, so to speak, and encourages more and more of those iron cannonballs to roll into our intestinal cells. It is just the plant-based iron, not that from meat, that is affected, but the effect is quite strong, with increases in iron absorption from two to four times and even greater in some cases.

Could taking extra vitamin C eventually increase your total iron load? Unfortunately, this important question is not fully resolved at the present time. Studies to date have either been inadequately designed or too small to really nail down the answer. We do know that as a person's iron stores increase, the percentage of plant-based iron (non-heme iron) that is absorbed decreases. While many scientists believe that this should eventually counteract the effect of vitamin C, others feel that this control mechanism is far from perfect and that it can be easily overridden, especially if vitamin C is taken over a long period of time.

The real danger is for people who have very high iron levels and begin taking large doses of vitamin C. Here we have complete agreement among iron experts.[19,20] Vitamin C exacerbates iron-induced damage to tissues, particularly in the heart, where it leads to a deadly form of heart disease called *congestive cardiomyopathy*. People with hemochromatosis, the inherited iron-overload disease, often develop this form of heart disease anyway, but vitamin C seems to accelerate the damage by shifting iron from dormant storage sites to the front lines of destruction.

In 1982, a group of doctors in Australia reported the tragic case of a twenty-nine-year-old male office worker who came into the hospital with a rapid heartbeat.[21] He had been feeling tired for two months, but prior to that he felt fine and was even able to play rugby competitively. For a year he had been taking 1000 milligrams of vitamin C a day and had been regularly drinking artificial orange juice containing even more of the vitamin. The doctors diagnosed severe heart failure but were unable to stabilize his condition: he died eight days after admission. From data collected prior to and after his death, the doctors were able to diagnose him as a hemochromatosis victim. (They subsequently found that two of his younger brothers also had the disease.) The doctors concluded the excessive vitamin-C intake was probably responsible for the patient's rapid deterioration.

This report as well as others in the medical literature over the past ten years have cast a new light on this popular vitamin. It is clear that diagnosed iron-overload patients should not take vitamin C. But, with a fifth or more of the American people taking vitamin C regularly, one has to wonder about the potential dangers for the hundreds of thousands of undiagnosed hemochromatosis victims who may be unknowingly putting themselves at risk. I also worry about the effects of excess vitamin C on people with even moderately high iron levels. Since iron may contribute to major killers such as heart disease and cancer, vitamin C could accelerate this destructive process by increasing iron absorption and exacerbating iron-induced tissue damage.

The concern that undiagnosed hemochromatosis victims could be harmed by vitamin C was one reason the 1980–1985 RDA Committee of the National Academy of Sciences tried to decrease the RDA for this vitamin from 60 milligrams a day to 40 milligrams for men and 30 for women.[19] While their main concern was that there was no good evidence that higher amounts were beneficial, these experts explicitly mentioned the possibility of iron toxicity from vitamin C. Unfortunately, the attempt to decrease the RDA was bulldozed by "pro–vitamin C" NAS staff members who rewrote these recommendations and, in 1990, issued the tenth edition of the RDAs with the RDA for vitamin C set back at its original value.[22]

How can you minimize vitamin C's effect on your iron levels yet still get enough of this important nutrient? Since C must be eaten with food or soon thereafter to enhance iron absorption, one solution is to try to eat foods rich in vitamin C, particularly citrus fruits, as snacks between meals. A refreshing glass of orange juice is good anytime; you do not have to have it with breakfast.

There is obviously a limit to the effectiveness of this measure. Throughout your day you are going to be eating other foods that are rich in vitamin C, such as tomatoes, broccoli, cauliflower, and various fruits, and there is no way you are going to prevent these foods from enhancing iron absorption. Vitamin C can even partially offset the protective effect of phytic acid in the intestines. And the most important factor is that you need the other invaluable nutrients in these foods. But nonetheless, by moving some of your citrus intake to snack times, you can depress vitamin C's bad effects on iron while still benefiting from its good properties.

If you think your diet is inadequate and you insist on taking vitamin C or multivitamin supplements, here are some guidelines you should follow:

- Don't take more than 100 percent of the RDA (60 milligrams).
- Try taking the supplements between meals to minimize the effect of iron absorption.

- Make sure you do not have hemochromatosis or excessively high iron levels before taking any vitamin C supplement. See Chapter 20 for more information on tests for high iron levels.

If You Like Tea or Coffee, Drink Some With Your Meals or Within the First Hour After You Eat

It is well known that tea and coffee, two of the most popular drinks in the world, can decrease the amount of plant-based iron absorbed from meals.[23-25] In developing countries, this is thought to contribute to iron deficiency, particularly in women. On the other hand, our well-fed, iron-rich population would be better off with less iron, and tea and coffee are helpful in this regard. These drinks have even been recommended to iron-overload patients.

Tea contains substantial quantities of tannic acid, a substance that latches on to iron in the stomach and intestines, reducing the amount available for absorption. Similar substances are present in coffee. While researchers have begun to focus on the health-promoting effects of these substances,[26] collectively called polyphenols, they have yet to test whether some of the beneficial effects stem from iron binding.

These substances are nearly as effective in reducing iron absorption as phytic acid, the iron-binding chemical in whole grains and legumes. Teas that have been tested, including Lipton's orange pekoe and pekoe-cut black tea and Twinings English breakfast tea, reduced iron absorption by 62–68 percent. Drip coffees—for example, Folger's and Gevalia, a Swedish brand—blocked iron uptake by 35–61 percent. Instant coffee (Taster's Choice from Nestlé) was even more effective (83 percent reduction). Researchers found that doubling the strength of the instant coffee caused further inhibition of iron absorption. Other beverages tested in these studies either did not have significant effects (water and Coca-Cola) or they *enhanced* iron absorption (alcohol and vitamin C–rich orange juice).[24,25]

One study showed that tea and coffee act to reduce iron absorption when they are given with meals or one hour after. No effect was seen when the beverages were consumed one hour prior to mealtime.[25]

The only other point you need to keep in mind when following this particular Iron Balance tip is that regular tea and coffee are potent drugs, and you should not get too much of them. The ill-effects due to excessive caffeine range from mild ones such as insomnia, anxiety attacks, indigestion, diarrhea, rapid heart-beat, and fibrocystic breast disease to more serious and even tragic events such as birth defects and a higher risk of miscarriage, stillbirths, and premature births. For these reasons, most authorities recommend limiting your caffeine intake to 300 milligrams a day, the equivalent of about two cups of coffee or four cups of tea. Pregnant women are advised to avoid caffeine altogether.

Though it has not been explicitly tested for effects on iron absorption, decaffeinated coffee should be about as good as regular coffee. Chemical analyses have shown that the magic substances in regular coffee that are responsible for decreased iron absorption are also present in decaffeinated brands, though sometimes in lower quantities. Caffeine-free teas, including herb teas, may also work, but they vary widely in their content of the iron-binding substances.

Do Not Cook in Iron Pots

Cooking food in cast iron pots, such as iron skillets or Dutch ovens, can increase the amount of iron in the food by three to a hundred times the original concentration.[27] Foods often help to leach iron from the pots. This is especially true of acidic foods, such as tomato sauce, where the acid assists in this process.

You would do well to take your iron pots out of commission. Perhaps you can use them as kitchen decorations, souvenirs of America's high-iron culinary past.

The Iron Balance Suggested Menu

Now you are ready to put these tips together into a workable daily meal plan. The suggested menu below gives you the foundation for a balanced low-fat, low-iron diet: it is up to you to adapt it to your tastes. As mentioned in the introduction to this chapter, you could consult several recent books, such as *Jane Brody's Good Food Book*, for recipes.[28,29]

With a few important differences, the Iron Balance menu is very similar to that recommended by the American Heart Association, the American Cancer Society, and other organizations. It is low in fat, cholesterol, and calories, and it is high in fiber. The important differences make the Iron Balance menu low on iron: I estimate that the daily iron intake would be in the range of 5 to 10 milligrams, far short of the excessive U.S. RDA for iron of 18 milligrams. If you stick to this menu or one similar to it, you should be able to lower your iron and cholesterol levels and perhaps even lose some weight.

The main features of the suggested menu are:

- One serving of meat per day at most, preferably fish or poultry.
- At least one serving of phytate-rich whole grains or legumes at *each* meal to minimize iron absorption.
- Citrus fruit or juice as between-meal snacks to minimize iron absorption while still supplying ample vitamin C.
- Optional tea or coffee to minimize iron absorption.
- No alcohol, or not more than three drinks per week.
- Plenty of fruits, vegetables, and low-fat or nonfat dairy products to round out your balanced diet.

SUGGESTED MENU
Breakfast

Whole-grain cereal, preferably bran, or bread, with no more than 25 percent of the RDA of iron (4.5 milligrams) per serving

Low-fat milk

Fruit

Coffee or tea (optional)

Mid-Morning Snack (optional)

Citrus fruit or juice

Lunch

Whole grain– or legume-based main course such as whole wheat pasta or bean salad

Vegetable or green salad

Low-fat milk or cottage cheese

Fruit

Coffee or tea (optional)

Mid-Afternoon Snack (optional)

Citrus fruit or juice

Dinner

Low-fat fish, turkey, or chicken dish

Whole-grain item such as rye or whole wheat bread; or peas, beans, or other legume dish

Two servings of vegetables, or vegetable and salad

Fruit

Coffee or tea (optional)

How Does the Iron Balance Menu Compare to Existing Diet Plans?

The names "Pritikin" and "Scarsdale" are etched into American diet culture. Whether it is for weight loss or overall health, Americans love a new diet craze. The question for now is, how do these diets stack up against the Iron Balance diet in terms of estimated iron intake?

Michele Fisher and Dr. Paul Lachance, nutritionists at Rutgers University in New Jersey, estimated the iron contents in a large number of popular diets in 1985.[30] In the table below, I have added my analysis of the Iron Balance menu and a few popular diets that were not included in the original study.[3,28,29,31-33] Keep in mind that these are crude estimates of iron content, not the total amount of iron actually absorbed from these diets. In addition, the amount of iron in most of the menus varies widely from day to day; I have reported the statistical ranges in the table.

You can see that the Iron Balance menu ranks in the low-iron category. This is due to the low meat content and the lack of iron-supplemented foods. In addition, the unique features of the Iron Balance menu, such as the inclusion of phytate-rich foods in every meal and the movement of citrus intake to snack times, may result in lower iron-absorption rates; the same cannot be said for the other diets listed. I also cannot speak for whether many of these diets are as balanced as the Iron Balance menu. The Fisher-Lachance study did indicate that many of them were low in several important nutrients.

Estimated Iron Content of Popular Diets

Diet	Range of Iron Content Per Day (milligrams)
Low-Iron Choices	
Iron Balance suggested menu	5.0–10.0
Richard Simmons	6.5–10.5
Scarsdale	7.5–12.5
Beverly Hills	5.5–17.5
Medium-Iron Choices	
Atkins	10.5–14.5
I Love America	10.5–15.0
Carbohydrate Craver's Basic	10.0–17.5
Carbohydrate Craver's Dense	11.5–16.5
Pritikin (700 calories)	12.5–15.5
American Heart Association (Step 1)	around 14.0
Stillman	9.0–21.5

Diet	Range of Iron Content Per Day (milligrams)
High-Iron Choices	
California (1200 calories)	9.0–24.0
American Heart Association (Step 2)	around 17.0
Jane Brody's Good Food Book (fall menu)	14.0–21.4
I Love New York	14.0–22.5
Controlling Cholesterol (Basic)	18.0–21.0
T-Factor	16.0–24.0
Pritikin (1200 calories)	17.5–23.5
Nutripoints	14.5–28.0
Dr. Berger's Immune Power Diet (women's menu)	17.2–25.5
California (2000 calories)	14.5–30.5
F-Plan	24.5–28.5

The Iron Balance Diet: A Good Start But Not a Cure-All

The low-fat, low-iron diet is a critical part of your new healthy life-style. You may have already begun to reduce the fat content in your diet; now you just have to add some "iron awareness" to your meal selection.

But if you truly want to "get the rust out" and minimize the possible effects of even moderately elevated iron levels, a good diet probably will not get you there fast enough. As you will read in the following chapter, the most efficient way to get rid of unwanted iron is to donate blood occasionally. Adding this new preventive measure to your low-fat, low-iron diet will make an unbeatable combination.

18

Donating Blood to Remove Excess Iron

When I describe the Iron Balance health plan to physicians I know, they are always a bit stunned by the notion of blood donation as a preventive measure to reduce the amount of excess iron in men and older women. While they understand the scientific premise behind the advantage of lower iron levels, the blood donation idea is too big a leap for most of them. "Are you really trying to bring back bloodletting?" they ask, referring to the often abused technique so popular in medicine before the twentieth century.

Occasional blood donation is probably the most controversial element of the Iron Balance Health Plan. While blood donation is widely recognized as being safe for almost everyone, the suggestion that it actually may be good for one's health can make a doctor's skin crawl. Doctors have little in common with those early men of medicine who relied largely upon superstition and brutish methods. The ancient physicians knew as much about the human body as today's butchers; they would try to drive out evil fluids from their patients by exhaustive bleeding, hurting rather than helping, in most cases. In contrast, doctors today are, by comparison, true miracle workers. Their detailed un-

215

derstanding of the human body, together with modern drugs and techniques, allows them to truly heal the sick rather than placate psychological needs. How could such a barbaric technique as bloodletting be useful in this brave new world of medicine?

Just as modern drugs are often found in ancient herbal remedies, I believe that the ancient technique of bloodletting, applied in a sophisticated manner to maintain lower iron levels, can become a useful and effective preventive measure. In this chapter, you will learn how blood donation is more effective than dietary measures in reducing iron levels. Blood donation is also the only preventive technique, aside from the occasional "walk-a-thon," that allows you to help others with a gift of life while doing something healthy for yourself. For the novice and those who want to know more about blood donation, I present a step-by-step account of what goes on when you decide to donate, including a description of health and age requirements, the processing of your blood, and the unique "donor's high" that people feel after it's all over.

But first, let's wipe off the cobwebs and take a close look at the barbaric use of bloodletting throughout history, and at the surprising recent acceptance of bloodletting as a standard therapeutic technique for certain diseases.

"Apply Ten Leeches and See Me in the Morning"

Bloodletting has been used as a therapeutic—but not preventive—technique from the beginning of recorded history. Perhaps the observation of bleeding from wounds or menstruation suggested the use of this technique to primitive civilizations. In South America, medicine men used bloodletting to draw out evil demons. But the most popular rationale for bloodletting was to restore the balance of the four "humors" or fluids: blood, mucus or phlegm, and the two types of bile, yellow and black. Many diseases were ascribed to an excess of blood that led to fever and other symptoms. The obvious solution was to reduce the amount of blood in the body.

Bloodletting became especially popular in the Middle Ages.

With the aid of astrology, special calendars were devised to determine optimal bleeding times. The exact technique that should be used—which veins to select, how much blood to draw—was hotly debated. A long brouhaha over bloodletting technique ensued in 1514 after Pierre Brissot, a Paris physician and medical professor, proclaimed that, contrary to the current tradition, blood should be drawn according to the age-old teachings of Hippocrates: near the site of disease rather than on the opposite side of the body. For this heresy, Brissot was banned by the French parliament and later chastised by Emperor Charles V of the Holy Roman Empire. Brissot's views won out in the end when one of Charles V's relatives died from bloodletting applied in the traditional, opposite-side fashion.

As bloodletting in France reached a peak in the 1830s, a shortage of bloodsucking leeches threatened the medical practice of the day. In the year 1833 alone, it was estimated that France imported 41.5 million leeches; at least 20 million a year were used for bloodletting throughout the 1830s. One prominent physician, François Broussais, was particularly nuts over the use of leeches for his patients, applying as many as ten to fifty at once to the stomach, head, and other sites, including the anus.

One medical historian speculated that the composer Frédéric Chopin, a tuberculosis victim, was fortunate to be treated at the time by Parisian doctors who were less bloodthirsty. As a result, Chopin lived until age thirty-nine, which enabled him to complete some of his most ambitious works for the piano. Mozart, on the other hand, was less fortunate; recent research indicates that he died from the effects of bloodletting administered to counter acute rheumatic fever.

Like primitive brews, concoctions, drugs, and other therapies, bloodletting was greatly misused by the ignorant medicine men of yore. Without question, bloodletting caused far less healing than it did misery and death. It is thought that the demise of our first president, George Washington, was hastened by copious bleeding on what would turn out to be the day of his death. The scientific evidence against bloodletting was first offered by Pierre Louis, the father of medical statistics, who shocked French medicine in 1840 with cold, hard numerical evidence that bloodletting was not a general panacea.[1-4]

Bloodletting Reconsidered

With the benefit of scientific hindsight, modern-day medical sleuths have hypothesized that, in some cases, bloodletting may have been helpful.[5] For example, it is feasible that bloodletting could reduce the severity of various bacterial infections, a major cause of death before the twentieth century. Frequent bleeding reduces iron levels, and, as described in Chapter 13, this in turn can reduce the growth of bacteria and other organisms which depend on iron. Of course, the ancient medicine man would have no knowledge of how to properly select patients who might benefit from this treatment. Nonetheless, the broad application of bloodletting may have spared at least a few lives every year.

Today, after a long period of disregard, bloodletting, also known as phlebotomy, has returned as a specific and often life-saving treatment for several diseases. The most important of these include:[6]

Hereditary hemochromatosis, the iron-overload disease. As discussed in Chapter 7, phlebotomy gets rid of excess iron and significantly prolongs the lives of hemochromatosis victims.

Polycythemia vera. This is a disease of the bone marrow that leads to the excessive production of blood cells. The blood becomes too thick to flow easily, and victims often suffer strokes or damage to a variety of tissues and organs. Before the use of phlebotomy, life expectancy after diagnosis was commonly 6 to 18 months. Nowadays, two to four phlebotomies a year, alone or in combination with drug therapy, extends the lives of these patients by eight to fifteen years.

Porphyria cutanea tarda, the "werewolf" disease. This disease, characterized by dark scars on the skin and excessive hair growth on the face and hands, is usually due to alcoholism. Less commonly, it can also stem from estrogen therapy, use of oral contraceptives, or from inherited factors. It has been thought that the werewolves of the Middle Ages were victims of this disease. Sunlight is known to trigger the appearance of the awful lesions; this presumably led the "werewolves" to shun the daylight and go out only at night. Scientists have noted that many of the victims of this disease also have iron overload. Their lesions and other symptoms do not reappear when they are treated with phlebotomy.

In addition to these three diseases, phlebotomy has also been used or at least mentioned for treatment of several other conditions, including pulmonary edema, high blood pressure, kidney disease, and iron overload resulting from kidney dialysis.

Can Blood Donation Improve Your Health?

Clearly, bloodletting has come full circle, from widespread acceptance to disfavor and back to acceptance again, if only for a few specific conditions. It is now a proven medical therapy, particularly when excess iron must be removed. While many doctors still view the technique as antiquated, it seems that bloodletting is here to stay.

With the growing body of evidence that even moderately elevated iron levels may be unhealthy, bloodletting may become an important *preventive* measure as well. The removal of iron-rich red blood cells stimulates the bone marrow to step up its production of these and other cells. Iron is drawn from storage sites in several organs for this purpose, thus lowering the general iron level in the body.

It has been known for years that blood donors have lower iron levels than nondonors. A review of four studies that examined the effect of blood donation on serum ferritin levels, the indicator for storage iron, found that men who donated regularly had total iron stores of about 470 milligrams, compared to 1240 milligrams for nondonors; regular blood donation by women dropped their iron levels from 450 to 250 milligrams.[7]

Over the years, several authors in the medical literature have speculated that blood donation could be a preventive measure, particularly as a defense against heart attacks. Early workers thought that blood donation would thin the blood and make it easier for the heart to pump, reducing stress on the heart and the risk of blood clots. However, these effects are not thought to be important.

In an important article published in 1981 in the British medical journal *Lancet*, Dr. Jerome Sullivan, a professor of pathology at the Medical University of South Carolina, first suggested that reducing iron levels through blood donation may be effective in reducing heart disease deaths.[8] The growing links between iron and heart disease as well as other chronic diseases suggest that blood donation might also be effective in preventing these illnesses. Unfortunately, there have been no studies to date that have adequately tested whether blood donation can prolong life. One preliminary Italian study did find a survival advantage of donors over nondonors.[9] Among people aged sixty-five to sixty-nine, for example, the death rate of donors was half that of nondonors. However, this relatively small study (332 donors and 399 nondonors) failed to take into account the fact that repeat donors may be a healthier lot compared to the general population. This selection bias occurs because only healthy people are allowed to donate.

Dr. Sullivan has pointed out that at the very least, the Italian study revealed that blood donation did not appear to be harmful. He has gone on to suggest several other study designs that would more accurately test whether blood donation is a life-saving measure.[10] At the time of this writing, he is currently discussing these ideas with the blood-banking community.

While many physicians have a certain distaste for blood-letting as preventive medicine, I believe that the weight of the evidence against iron will convince enough of them to permit proper, large-scale studies of the effect of blood donation on health. What you must ask yourself is whether you are willing to risk living the high-iron life-style for an indefinite period of time while these studies are conducted and their results debated. It could be quite a long haul. And with the entrenched views that iron is safe and bloodletting is barbaric, it is definitely uphill.

If you have never donated blood, consider doing so now. The most important reason to donate—to help others—has always been there. The possible health benefits are an attractive bonus. As you will read in the following pages, blood donation is the fastest route to iron balance. Let's see how it works on a typical member of our high-iron society.

How Can Tom Reduce His Iron Level?

Tom is that typical meat-and-potatoes guy you met in Chapter 14, who scored pretty high on the self-test: the test predicted that he had 1790 milligrams of storage iron, far more than he needs. Can he reduce his iron level by the Iron Balance dietary measures alone? The answer is yes, but it is going to take a long, long time.

Let's do what scientists call a "back-of-the-envelope calculation," a crude estimate. To drop his iron level to around 400 milligrams, just inside the safe range, Tom needs to lose roughly 1400 milligrams of iron. Let's say he follows the Iron Balance dietary recommendations to a T and restricts his intake to around 10 milligrams of iron a day. If we assume that 5 percent of that dietary iron is actually absorbed, Tom will get about .5 milligram a day. With typical iron losses for men of 1 milligram per day from sweat, urine, and the shedding of intestinal cells, Tom will be losing about .5 milligram of iron per day from his iron stores. *At this rate, it will take him seven years or more to reach the safe 400-milligram level!*

As you can see, the Iron Balance diet is good at preventing additional iron buildup, but it cannot remove excess iron efficiently. Likewise, as you will learn in the following chapter, the other preventive measure to shed excess iron—exercise—also works quite slowly.

The only way Tom can reduce his rust level fairly rapidly is by donating blood. Each pint of Tom's blood contains around 236 milligrams of iron in the form of hemoglobin, the oxygen-carrying substance inside red blood cells. (A pint of blood from a woman contains slightly less iron, about 213 milligrams.) Each time a pint of blood is removed, this same quantity of iron is removed from its storage sites and put to work as newly formed hemoglobin. Tom can repeat this process as often as every eight weeks if he chooses, or he can spread it out over a longer period. In any case, *he can easily get rid of 1400 milligrams of unwanted, excess iron by donating six times over one to two years*. In Chapter 20, I'll show you how to figure out the number of blood donations you need to undergo to get iron-balanced.

Compared to other preventive measures, such as lowering

cholesterol levels by diet and/or drugs, blood donation is marvelously efficient. For example, my iron levels dropped over 20 percent after donating only one unit of blood. In contrast, many people have a difficult time reducing their cholesterol level even 5 to 10 percent over the course of a year or longer.

Another unique aspect of blood donation is that you are helping others while you are helping yourself. As he goes through his "derusting" process, Tom will have the pleasure of providing blood to many people who need it.

Donating to a Precious National Resource

Blood is an invaluable resource for our health care system. Whole blood, red cells, and other blood constituents are desperately needed for a wide range of patients undergoing surgery, treatment of injuries, or other life-saving procedures. In 1987, 11.6 million units of whole blood or red cells were transfused in the U.S. (A unit of whole blood is slightly less than a pint.) This is equivalent to the use of one unit roughly *every three seconds*.

The acquired immune deficiency syndrome (AIDS) epidemic has drastically changed the practice of blood banking and transfusion. In the early 1980s, it was discovered that the AIDS virus could be spread through blood transfusion. This prompted a herculean and largely successful effort on the part of the blood banks to ensure the safety of our blood supply with rigorous testing of each donated pint of blood. (Many people still harbor the mistaken belief that one can get AIDS by *donating* blood. This is impossible, as a sterilized, nonreusable needle is used for each blood donor.) The fear of contaminated blood has also led doctors to use blood more sparingly; the total units transfused each year in the U.S. has actually begun to decline.

Nonetheless, the demand for blood remains high. The three organizations in charge of blood collections, the American Red Cross, the American Association of Blood Banks, and the Council of Community Blood Centers, still must work hard to sustain the supply, particularly when a higher number of potential donors are now turned away because of possible exposure to the

AIDS virus. Donor recruitment, often using a "bloodmobile," has become of paramount importance to blood banks, and many new groups of people, such as large numbers of healthy older citizens, have become targets of these efforts. One blood bank near Tampa, Florida, even goes so far as to drive its mobile unit to a local nudist camp each summer!

Regional shortages, particularly during holiday periods, often threaten our blood supply. New York City is hardest hit, requiring the importation of roughly three hundred thousand units of blood each year, much of it from Europe. Other metropolitan areas that cannot meet their needs include Chicago, Boston, Los Angeles, and Miami. Even if you do not live in these cities, your donation can help alleviate shortages around the country, since blood is shipped to where it is needed most.[11-14]

The Gift

If the goal of lowering your iron levels is one reason you choose to donate blood, don't lose sight of the fact that it helps others as well. The inclusion of blood donation in the Iron Balance Health Plan makes it the only altruistic health plan in existence.

Blood is a gift like no other. Richard Titmuss, the author of an important book on blood donation and blood banking, *The Gift Relationship: From Human Blood to Social Policy*, described it best:[15]

> In terms of the free gift of blood to unnamed strangers there is no formal contract, no legal bond, no situation of power, domination, constraint or compulsion, no sense of shame or guilt, no gratitude imperative, no need for a reward or a return gift. They are acts of free will; of the exercise of choice; of conscience without shame.

It is interesting to hear some of the reasons people give the "gift of life." Titmuss's book described a 1967 survey of 3800 British donors who responded to the question, "Could you say why you *first* decided to become a blood donor?" Some of the answers were unforgettable. Here are what a few of the respondents actually wrote:

"Knowing I might be saving somebody's life." (Forty-year-old woman who has donated ten times in her life.)

"You can't get blood from supermarkets and chain stores. Sick people can't get out of bed to ask you for a pint to save their life, so I came forward to help somebody who needs blood." (Twenty-three-year-old woman; four donations.)

"No man is an island." (Thirty-six-year-old man; twenty-one donations.)

"I thought it was just a small way to help people—as a blind person other opportunities are limited." (Forty-nine-year-old-man, a piano tuner; twenty-six donations.)

"Some unknown person gave blood to save my wife's life." (Forty-three-year-old man; fifty-six donations.)

"No money to spare [for charity]. Plenty of blood to spare." (Thirty-five-year-old man, a painter and decorator; nineteen donations.)

A few other people had different reasons, such as a personal appeal from someone else—a man responded, "A pretty young nurse walked round the factory I was working in"—or post-donation treats—"To get a good cup of tea."

Whatever their reasons, most people experience some form of emotional gratification after donating, such as heightened self-esteem or a sense of feeling special. I will discuss this "donor's high" later in this chapter.

The Blood Donation Experience

With only 6 percent of Americans providing the blood for the entire country, it is clear that a lot of people have either never been asked to donate or are frightened of the idea. I was a member of the "cowards anonymous club" for many years, having been deathly afraid of needles for as long as I can remember. When I learned how blood donation could reduce my iron levels, I decided it was time to give it a try. Having conquered my irrational fears, I must tell you novices out there that it's no big deal.

For those of you who have never donated blood or would like to know more about the process, the following sections take you through it step by step. The entire blood donation procedure, including a health history and a physical, takes only about an hour.

Choosing the Type of Blood Donation

If you would like to reduce your iron levels, you should donate whole blood, which contains the iron-rich red blood cells. This is by far the most common form of blood donation. Other forms of blood donation include *plasmapheresis*, in which only the plasma—the liquid part of blood, not the cells—is taken, and *hemapheresis*, in which cells other than red blood cells are removed.

You may also hear the term *autologous donation*. This is an increasingly popular option for people with upcoming surgery who are allowed to predonate their own blood, the safest kind for a transfusion, in the three to four weeks prior to the scheduled surgery. (Blood can be refrigerated for only six weeks.) The amount a person can predonate in this short period of time is limited so that the patient doesn't become anemic. However, the commercial availability of a special, genetically engineered human hormone known as *erythropoietin*, which speeds up the production of red cells, may soon allow people to set aside all they need.[16]

Finding a Place to Donate

Choose a nonprofit institution such as a nearby hospital or local American Red Cross donor center.

Before You Donate

Most centers recommend eating a light meal no more than two hours before donating.

Age Requirements

Current policy states that blood donation is restricted to adults eighteen years of age and older. With a signed consent form from a parent or guardian, seventeen-year-olds can also donate.

People sixty-five or older used to be required to bring a note from a physician certifying that they were fit to donate. After a recent Harvard Medical School study showed that blood banks were missing out on some good, older donors, this policy has been changed so that elderly donors are accepted at the discretion of the medical director at the donor center.[16, 17]

Weight Requirements

Because of the size of the standard unit of blood, you must be at least 110 pounds (50 kilograms) so that the amount of blood withdrawn does not affect you. In countries where people are naturally smaller, for example Japan, the standard amount of blood collected is much less than the pint collected in Western countries. If you are less than 110 pounds and would like to donate blood, you will have to find a donor center that will accept smaller amounts of blood.[18]

Health Requirements

After registering with an official at the donor center, you will complete a confidential health history form. American Red Cross centers will examine the following health factors:[16]

Condition	Can I Donate?
Active allergies, no symptoms today	Yes
Active allergies, symptoms today	No
AIDS, or AIDS-related complex, or a positive test for anti-HIV	No
Angina	No
Arthritis	Yes
Asthma, no symptoms today	Yes
Asthma, symptoms today	No
Blood transfusion, *more* than 6 months ago	Yes
Blood transfusion, *less* than 6 months ago	No
Cancer, skin or cervical	Yes
Cancer, other than skin or cervical cancer	No
Cold; exposure to a cold but feel well with no symptoms	Yes
Cold, active	No
Diabetes, no insulin use	Yes
Diabetes, with insulin use	No
Epilepsy or seizures, controlled by medication; no episode within last year	Yes
Fever	No
Flu; exposure to flu but feel well with no symptoms	Yes
Flu, active	No
Heart attack	No
Hepatitis, household contact; exposure to hepatitis *more* than 6 months ago	Yes
Hepatitis, viral	No
High blood pressure, controlled with medication	Yes
Jaundice as a newborn	Yes
Jaundice, at present time	No
Malaria:	
• Residence in malarial area *more* than 3 years ago	Yes
• Travel in malarial area with antimalaria drugs *more* than 3 years ago	Yes

Condition	Can I Donate?
• Travel in malarial area without antimalaria drugs *more* than 6 months ago	Yes
Medications:	
• Antibiotics	
• Injected antibiotics, *more* than 4 weeks ago	Yes
• Oral antibiotics, *more* than 2 days ago	Yes
• For acne	Yes
• Accutane for acne	No
• Allergy pills	Yes
• Aspirin	Yes
• Birth control pills	Yes
Mononucleosis; exposure to mono but feel well with no symptoms	Yes
Mononucleosis, with symptoms	No
Pregnancy	No
Pregnancy, recent; postpartum by 6 weeks, vaginal delivery	Yes
Pregnancy, recent; caesarean section *more* than 3 months ago	Yes
Rubella vaccine (German measles), *more* than 4 weeks ago	Yes
Strep; exposure to strep but feel well with no symptoms	Yes
Strep, with symptoms	No
Stroke	No
Surgery; major surgery *more* than 3 months ago	Yes
Surgery; healed minor surgery	Yes
Tooth extraction, *more* than 3 days ago	Yes
Tuberculosis; 2 years after full recovery	Yes
Vaccines: *more* than 2 weeks since vaccine for measles, mumps, polio, smallpox, or yellow fever	Yes

The Health Exam

You will have your temperature, blood pressure, and pulse taken to make sure you are in good health. In addition, two biochemical tests will be performed on a single sample of blood obtained from a simple finger puncture. The first test is for the level of hemoglobin, the oxygen-carrying substance in your blood. The test used is not the best, but it is fast. If hemoglobin values are below 12.5 grams per 100 milliliters of blood for men and 12 grams per 100 milliliters for women, another more accurate test is usually run to see if you are truly anemic. This test, known as the hematocrit, actually measures the number of red cells in your blood. (A recent study indicated that a second blood sample should be taken for this measurement; otherwise too many people are falsely deterred from donating.) If this result is also low, you will have to try donating another time.

The second test measures the amount of a liver enzyme, *alanine aminotransferase* (ALT), in the blood. A high level of this substance signals liver damage. Since liver damage could be due to the hepatitis virus, which can be passed on to the blood recipient, potential donors with high ALT results will be deterred.

The Donation

A staff person will escort you to a reclining chair and clean the arm of your choice (usually the left arm for right-handed people and vice versa). A sterile, nonreusable needle is used to draw blood from a vein in your arm. As your donation begins, you will feel a slight pinch.

The staff member will stay with you and make sure you are feeling all right. If you are like me, you might feel a little faint—this is largely psychological. If so, just ask for a cool towel for your forehead or for a fan to blow cool air right at you. Talking to the nurse will help as well. These measures have kept a champion fainter—me!—from ever going down for the count while donating. Also, keep in mind that sensations such as these are more mild in subsequent donations.

Your donation will be over in about ten minutes.

What to Do After the Donation

After you have donated, you will relax in a special room for ten or fifteen minutes. Drink plenty of juice or other liquids to replace the fluids taken from your body and help yourself to the snacks provided. While the vast majority of people have no problem returning to their normal activities after donating, most centers recommend the following commonsense precautions:

1. Do not smoke for at least half an hour after donating blood.
2. Have a good meal after donating blood.
3. Leave the bandage in place for a few hours.
4. You may resume most normal activities after donating blood, but you should preferably avoid strenuous arm work or exercise for the rest of the day, as it could cause your needle site to bleed.
5. If any bleeding occurs at the needle site, raise your arm and apply light pressure directly to the bleeding until it stops.
6. If a bruise develops at a needle site some time after the procedure, pressure with an ice pack will help in the early stages. Later, a bruise will be slightly sore for about a week. If it bothers you at this stage, hot packs will speed up its disappearance.

How You Will Feel After the Donation: The "Donor's High"

After you donate, you'll feel great! Many donors experience a warm glow or sense of well-being after donating. Scientists have documented this elation response, the "donor's high," and some studies indicate that it intensifies with subsequent donations. In other words, the donor becomes "addicted" to helping others.[19]

These studies have also focused on anxiety felt *before* donation. This anxiety steadily decreases with the number of blood donations: the old pros exhibit virtually no anxiety, even though they still feel the "high" afterward.

What Happens to Your Blood

After passing the rigorous testing for infectious diseases, your blood will be separated into the various components different patients need. It usually will be available for someone who needs it a day or two after you donate.

While it is possible that your blood could be shipped to a community with a temporary shortage, it is more likely that it will be used right away in your metropolitan area or county. A recent *Reader's Digest* article told how the blood of Cecelia Feick, a twenty-nine-year-old housewife in Newport News, Virginia, was used in her community.[20] Various amounts of her anonymous gift, unit E29277, went to three grateful patients: a twenty-three-year-old insulation foreman who had inhalation burns, as well as burns over 75 percent of his body; a ninety-two-year-old woman who came to the hospital after experiencing fainting spells and strokelike symptoms, and who had internal bleeding and anemia; a man who needed coronary bypass surgery. This man was later quoted as saying, "I've donated over two gallons of blood in my day. Thank God somebody else's blood was there to backstop me when I needed it."

The article concluded, "They all owe their lives to the simple kindness of a stranger."

Answers to Common Questions About Blood Donation

How Often Can I Donate?

Regulations prohibit people from donating more than once every eight weeks. This is to prevent you from becoming temporarily anemic. If you stick to the same donor center, the staff will be able to keep track of the dates you donate and prevent you from donating too frequently. If you want to donate at a different center, make sure you know the date of your most recent donation.

Be sure to read Chapter 20 for instructions on how to determine the number of blood donations you need to make to get iron-balanced.

Is Blood Donation Safe?

Yes! Mild reactions such as fainting are extremely rare: they occur in less than 1 percent of blood donors. More serious reactions, such as vomiting, convulsions, or heart attack, are exceedingly rare.

Can I Get Paid for Donating Blood?

The only way to get paid for donating today is to go to a commercial plasma blood bank which pays eight to twenty-five dollars for each donation. Plasma is a source of important pharmaceutical products.

You will not reduce your iron levels by this type of donation, however, since only plasma is taken from your system, and none of the iron-rich red cells.

I would advise you to give your blood to nonprofit centers, such as your local hospital. If these blood banks have extra plasma, they can sell it to pharmaceutical companies and generate some revenue to help defray their operating costs.

The reason blood banks no longer pay donors is that it led to too many donations by unhealthy donors, especially those more likely to have hepatitis or other diseases.

19

One More Reason to Exercise

You can view exercise as a third tool against iron accumulation. Though not as effective as diet and blood donation, exercise can reduce your iron levels. Of course, you already have plenty of reasons to get out and sweat a little: it's good for your heart, your mind, and your sense of well-being, and it's fun. The possibility that exercise can help you become iron-balanced is icing on the cake.

Living Longer With Exercise

A number of studies have indicated that people who are more physically active live longer than sedentary folks. The latest study, performed by the Institute for Aerobics Research in Dallas, examined the fitness level, as determined by a treadmill test, and the mortality of over 13,000 men and women for an average of eight years.[1] The researchers, including Dr. Kenneth Cooper, the pioneer of the aerobics movement, found that fit individuals lived significantly longer than sedentary folks. The groups of people who were more fit, from the walkers to the more intense five-mile-a-day runners, all enjoyed reductions in both heart disease and cancer deaths.

While the large difference in mortality between the sedentary group and the group at the next highest fitness level was the most important finding of the study, there did appear to be some marginal gains in longevity in the higher fitness groups. This was especially true for women. Other studies have not shown an advantage for more athletic individuals. Further research will be required to see if the gains in longevity from more intense forms of exercise are worth the time and effort.

Can Traditional Reasons Explain the Magic of Exercise?

Most researchers believe that there may be a number of reasons that exercise is beneficial. Exercise may prevent heart disease by making the heart stronger and the coronary arteries larger and healthier. Exercise increases the amount of protective, or "good," cholesterol in the blood and reduces blood pressure and weight. It may also reduce stress and inhibit the clotting action of the blood. All these changes are for the better, and they alone should convince you to exercise.

But are these effects sufficient to explain the effectiveness of exercise in protecting the heart? Many of the changes in these important factors are relatively small. For example, one study found that improvements in blood pressure and cholesterol composition accounted for only 10 percent of exercise-related reductions in heart disease deaths.[2] And researchers have not yet shown that the other suggested effects, such as the decrease in the clotting ability of the blood, are responsible for the remaining reductions in mortality.

Why exercise would protect against cancer is even a greater mystery at this time. One plausible reason has been offered in the case of colon cancer: since exercise stimulates bowel activity, this would reduce the exposure of the bowel to harmful chemicals and may decrease the incidence of this one form of cancer.[3] But what about all the other types of cancer?

A more general explanation is that exercise stimulates the immune system to attack and destroy tumor cells. However, both stimulation *and* suppression of the immune system have been detected in people who have just exercised.[4,5]

There's another problem with these conventional explanations of how exercise reduces deaths from heart disease and cancer: not only are many of them insufficient and unproven, but they are also, in a way, at odds with one another. For example, from what we are beginning to learn about heart disease, there is reason to believe that the stimulation of the immune system, while protecting against cancer, may actually exacerbate the "hardening of the arteries" that leads to heart attacks. Immune-system cells called *macrophages* are known to be involved in this damaging process.

Another example is the effect of improved blood circulation, which, while protecting against heart disease, could stimulate tumor growth. A tumor cell's ability to grow and spread lethally throughout the body is intimately dependent upon its lifeline, the blood supply, and anything that enhances the delivery of oxygen and nutrients could increase its chances for success.

The Iron Hypothesis

The search for a unified mechanism to account for the protection exercise provides against both heart disease and cancer prompted me to examine the effect of exercise on iron levels.[6-8] Iron may play a role in the development of both diseases, and if iron levels were reduced by exercise, this would provide a more general explanation for the beneficial effects of this popular preventive regimen. As I quickly found out, the scientific literature is full of reports stating that exercise reduces iron levels. Let's look at some of the evidence.

Exercise "Gets the Rust Out"

The effects of exercise on iron metabolism have come largely from studies of athletes, particularly long-distance runners, in whom the changes have been easy to detect. The majority of these studies show that many athletes do have lower iron levels, even to the point where it can adversely affect their performance. This actually happened to Alberto Salazar, a world champion long-distance runner, who suffered from iron deficiency in 1983. Once the problem was corrected, he was able to qualify for the 1984 U.S. Olympic team.[9]

It's true that exercise places some demands on iron stores. Training is thought to increase the concentration of many iron-containing substances throughout the body, most of which are involved in transporting oxygen to muscles or in energy production. But this creates only a temporary demand on iron reserves; after a few weeks, an equilibrium is reached and little additional iron is required.

Over the long term, however, exercise actually decreases the amount of storage iron in the body.[10,11] This iron is not utilized for any special purpose—it is simply lost from the body, as described below. As a result, many athletes have low readings of serum ferritin, the best indicator for determining iron stores.

There appear to be three possible pathways for exercise-induced iron loss:

1. *Gastrointestinal bleeding.* Several studies have detected an increase in the amount of hemoglobin iron in the feces after an athletic event. Though not understood at the present time, researchers think that this bleeding is somehow related to either the lack of oxygen in the intestines during exercise or repetitive jarring of the internal organs. Iron losses through this mechanism can be as high as .25 to .6 milligram a day, or, if a person runs four times a week, 50 to 125 milligrams a year.

2. *Loss of hemoglobin iron in the urine.* Hemolysis, the destruction of red blood cells, is known to occur with strenuous exercise. This leads to the liberation of free hemoglobin, which is then excreted by the kidneys, resulting in a net loss of iron. The damage to the red cells may be due to increased body temperature or to bumps and bruises on the cell wall from the increased

circulatory rate, or to mechanical force, such as when the foot strikes the ground or when muscular action compresses tiny blood vessels. The amount of iron lost through this pathway can be .2 milligram a day, or roughly 40 milligrams a year.

3. *Loss of iron through sweat.* Iron is present in sweat in varying amounts. As much as one to three quarts of sweat can be lost in many forms of athletic activity. The loss of one quart would lead to an iron loss of roughly .15 milligram a day, or 30 milligrams a year.

An additional reason why athletes may have lower iron stores is that they appear to absorb less iron from the diet. In one study iron-deficient runners absorbed 16 percent of the iron in a test meal compared to 30 percent for iron-deficient nonrunners.[10] Researchers do not know why this occurs.

As you can see, it is quite easy for an athlete to reduce his or her iron stores by 100–200 milligrams each year. What about the rest of us who exercise less strenuously? This is an area where considerably more research must be done. One would expect that the iron losses from fitness-type exercise would be smaller than that from athletic training. However, the only good study to date, performed at the University of Illinois, suggests that significant reductions in iron levels can take place.[12] The iron levels in twenty-four nonathletic women were followed during a thirteen-week aerobic calisthenics class that met four times a week. After the sixth week, their average iron level, as estimated by serum ferritin measurements, dropped by 50 milligrams. However, no further change was detected over the remaining seven weeks.

Exercise May Also Move Iron Into Safe Storage

In addition to the actual loss of iron from the body, it is possible that exercise may also stimulate a repackaging of cellular iron for safer storage. This hypothesis is based on recent advancements in our understanding of the cellular effects of exercise.

Exercise is known to kick off a chain of chemical events in the body, including the release of hormones and other substances.[13,14] The "runner's high," for example, results from the release of certain brain chemicals. Scientists have recently discoverd that one of the substances released, a protein called *interleukin-1*, is a sort of "master molecule" that orchestrates a number of biochemical effects in the body, particularly in response to invasion by foreign organisms. Since high iron levels would encourage the growth of these organisms, one of the functions of the "master molecule" is to cause a decrease in the availability of iron in the blood. It does this by stimulating the production of ferritin, the "storage bin" for iron, which grabs any stray iron atoms and safely sequesters them away.[15-19] If exercise encourages iron storage the same way infection does, then over time we could expect that physical activity, even moderate forms, could lead to a much healthier situation, where iron is kept in its place and not allowed to roam free.

Why would exercise, one of the most natural and healthy activities, lead to a chain of events similar to that triggered by infection? Scientists have not solved this one yet, though they have speculated that damage to muscle fibers, even if subtle, could stimulate a repair response that includes the same chain of events that follows infection. It is also possible that the body recognizes exercise as a form of stress, resulting in the release of "stress hormones" and other substances that also lead to the release of the "master molecule."

Why Wait to Begin?

By now you have more than enough evidence demonstrating the benefits of exercise. Along with diet and occasional blood donation, physical activity may help maintain low iron levels while keeping you fit.

If you have not already begun to exercise, today is a good day to start. You can begin with brisk, thirty-minute walks at least three or four times a week. If you want to graduate to more strenuous activities, check with your doctor first, particularly if you are over forty years of age.

Keep in mind that most of the health gains accrue from moving out of the lazy, sedentary group and into the active set. Once in this group, it is questionable whether additional exercise is that beneficial. In *Dr. Dean Ornish's Program for Reversing Heart Disease*, the author calculates that strenuous exercise, say regular five-mile runs, may add up to two years to your life, but one and a half years of that is time that exercise and its preparations take out of your busy schedule.[20] The best advice is: keep active, but keep it fun!

If you need additional information to get your exercise program going, try Dr. Ornish's book or Dr. Kenneth Cooper's *The Aerobics Program for Total Well-Being*.

20

Putting It All Together

Now it's time to put the Iron Balance Health Plan to work for you. This chapter includes an easy five-step plan to start trimming your iron levels today. It also shows you how to estimate the number of times you should donate blood to get iron-balanced and stay that way. Later in the chapter I will show you how the Iron Balance Health Plan has worked for me.

Five Easy Steps to Iron Balance

Step 1. Eat Right

This is definitely something you can begin today if you have not already. Bypass that juicy steak at the restaurant, throw away those iron-containing supplements, and eat more high-fiber foods. Follow the recommendations in Chapter 17, but don't be too hard on yourself. Remember, if you start out hating a new diet, it is not going to last too long. If you are out with friends and want to celebrate, leave your new "iron awareness" at home and try to make up for it the next day.

Also, try not to forget what you probably already know about how to choose low-fat foods. The Iron Balance dietary recommendations will help you choose modest amounts of lean meats, but you also should keep away from fatty foods, choose low-fat or nonfat dairy products, and stay away from rich desserts. I have been living the low-fat, low-iron life-style for some time now, and it has kept my cholesterol level quite low: my latest reading was 127 milligrams per deciliter, about two-thirds that of most men my age.

Step 2. Get at Least a Moderate Amount of Exercise

As you read in the last chapter, exercise is not the most important part of the Iron Balance Health Plan, but it may help keep your iron levels down while it enhances your health and fitness.

Step 3. Donate Blood Once as Soon as You Have a Break in Your Schedule

For the 94 percent of Americans that have never donated blood, there is no need to procrastinate. Make the time to help someone out with your "gift of life" as soon as your schedule permits. If you were deterred from a donor center earlier in your life, try again. And if you are scared, just remember: it's no big deal. You've given blood samples probably dozens of times at your doctor's office. Blood donation is not much different.

I recommend that you donate only once until you have the results from a complete blood-iron analysis from your doctor (step 4). If you want to donate again before you get the results from the blood test, it's okay: the donor center will perform a satisfactory health exam and make sure you can spare the pint. But to be on the safe side, it's best to be patient and make sure your iron levels are high enough to warrant a second donation. For many people, one donation might be enough to get them iron-balanced.

Step 4. Get a Complete Blood-Iron Analysis From Your Doctor

Make an appointment with your doctor for a routine checkup and insist on the following blood-iron tests:

- serum ferritin
- serum iron
- total iron-binding capacity (also known as TIBC)

Your doctor may claim that he or she cannot justify these tests and may not be able to get reimbursed for them from your insurance company or health program. If this is the case, you can either change doctors or insist that you want the information and will pay for the tests yourself. (They can cost less than a routine visit to your dentist. In 1990, cost estimates ranged from $26.00 to $75.00.)

The first of the tests, the serum ferritin test, will indicate how much excess iron you have stored away in your body. Multiplying the result by ten will give you an estimate of your iron stores in units of milligrams. You will use this result in the next section. (You should be aware that the serum ferritin test is not perfect: the result can be falsely high, independent of the true iron level, for people with acute bacterial infections, rheumatoid arthritis, inflammatory bowel disease, liver disease, and certain forms of cancer. Other test results will allow your doctor to rule out these conditions.)

The other two tests, the serum iron test and the TIBC test, will allow you and your doctor to assess whether or not you have hemochromatosis, the hereditary iron-overload disease. *To be most accurate, both of these tests should be performed on blood withdrawn after you have fasted overnight.* Whether or not you have hemochromatosis can be determined by your transferrin saturation level: the percentage of the iron-binding capacity on the blood protein called transferrin, the "wheelbarrow" for iron, that has already been filled. Transferrin saturation can be calculated as follows:

$$\frac{\text{Serum iron result}}{\text{TIBC result}} \times 100 = \text{Transferrin saturation}$$

Transferrin saturation results of greater than 62 percent for men or 50 percent for women indicate that hemochromatosis may be present. If you fit into this category, you should insist on further evaluation by a specialist, preferably a hematologist, gastroenterologist, or internist. If the diagnosis is confirmed, you should begin bloodletting treatments (phlebotomy) immediately to remove the excess iron. Your blood relatives should also be screened for the disease.

Step 5. *Continue Donating Blood to Maintain Low Iron Levels*

The following table shows you how to get rid of excess iron within a year or two using blood donation. Your goal is to reduce your total iron stores to around 100–400 milligrams. For best results, use your actual serum ferritin measurement to estimate your present iron level. Then use the table as a guide to determine the number of blood donations you need to reach the 100–400 milligram range. Remember, *do not donate more than once every eight weeks*. If you stick to the same donor center, they will make sure you don't.

You can also use the table to see roughly where you stand after taking the Iron-Risk-Level Self-Test in Chapter 14. The score from the self-test is a crude approximation of your estimated iron stores.

After getting down to 100–400 milligrams of storage iron, you can stay roughly within this range or very near it by eating right and donating blood occasionally. How often should you donate? If you follow the Iron Balance diet closely, one blood donation a year is probably good enough. Otherwise, two donations a year may be needed.

Keep in mind that these estimates are quite crude. It is difficult to estimate how much iron you will be absorbing from your diet. This is particularly true when iron stores are low: the percentage of dietary iron that is absorbed increases by different amounts for different individuals.

Number of Blood Donations Required to Get Iron-Balanced

Iron Risk Level	Serum Ferritin Measurement[a]	× 10 =	Estimated Iron Stores (in milligrams)	Number of Initial Blood Donations[b]
Low	0–40		0–400	0
Intermediate	41–62		410–620	1
	63–84		630–840	2
High	85–106		850–1060	3
	107–128		1070–1280	4
	129–150		1290–1500	5
	151–172		1510–1720	6
Very High	173–194		1730–1940	7
	195–216		1950–2160	8
	217–238		2170–2380	9
	239–260		2390–2600	10
	261–282		2610–2820	11
	over 282		over 2820	12

[a]In units of nanograms per milliliter or micrograms per liter of blood serum.
[b]These should be spread out over one to two years. *Please remember that you should not donate more frequently than once every eight weeks!*

For these reasons, I recommend that you repeat steps 4 and 5 periodically, say every two to four years. This way you will know your serum ferritin level and total iron stores, and if your iron level has bumped up a little, you can more accurately estimate how many blood donations you might need to get back down to the 100–400 milligram range.

Your Iron Balance Diary

It is a good idea to keep a record of your blood donations and your test results, particularly your serum ferritin tests and your estimates of total iron stores. You will be able to follow your progress, and if you should move or change donor centers, you will know when you last gave blood. You can also record other test results from your doctor's appointments, such as your hemoglobin level, hematocrit (red-blood-cell concentration), cholesterol level, and your Iron-Risk-Level Self-Test score. The latter can be taken after each blood donation.

At the end of the book, you will find the Iron Balance Diary, a convenient place to store this information. You can take a look at my diary in the next section if you would like to see an example.

The Author As Guinea Pig

I started the Iron Balance Health Plan in the summer of 1989. I made gradual changes in my diet, and I started donating blood and keeping track of my test results. My Iron Balance diary is shown on the next page.

I had my serum ferritin level measured before I began the program and after each blood donation so that I could show you how effective blood donation is in removing excess iron. (You won't need to follow your own iron level so closely.) As I mentioned in Chapter 14, my self-test score of 800 milligrams was not too far from the estimate of 880 milligrams that I calculated from my first serum ferritin measurement of 88 units. This amount of excess iron is normal for American men in my age group.

As you can see from my diary, I do not appear to have iron-overload disease, since my transferrin saturation level was 22.6 percent, far lower than the 62 percent cutoff for men with this disease.

In Figure 20-2, you can see how my iron level dropped once I started donating blood. It fell from 880 to 590 milligrams after the first donation; from 590 to 330 milligrams after the second; and from 330 to 110 milligrams after the third. These results were similar to my self-test scores, which decreased from 800 to 600 to 400 and finally to 200. Though it is a very crude estimate, the self-test worked pretty well for me.

The IRON BALANCE Diary

Date	Blood Donation	Blood Test	Serum Ferritin Result x 10 = (ng/ml or µg/l)	Estimated Iron Stores (mg)	Comments or Other Test Results
7/31/89		X	88 x 10 = 880		
					SELF-TEST SCORE = 800 mg
					SERUM IRON = 80 MICROGRAM/100 ml
					TIBC = 354 MICROGRAM/100 ml
					TRANSFERRIN SATURATION =
					$\frac{80}{354} \times 100 = 22.6\%$
8/3/89	X				
9/21/89		X	59 x 10 = 590		SELF-TEST = 600 mg
9/28/89	X				
11/14/89		X	33 x 10 = 330		SELF-TEST = 400 mg
4/3/90	X				
5/25/90		X	11 x 10 = 110		SELF-TEST = 200 mg
					HEMOGLOBIN = 14.3 g/100 ml

Figure 20-1. The author's Iron Balance diary. I had a serum ferritin blood test run before donating blood. The result—88 units—converts to an estimated level of iron stores of 880 milligrams. This agrees quite well with my self-test score of 800 milligrams of iron. The other entries you see for July 31, 1989, are two additional blood tests from the same sample of my blood, the serum iron and total iron-binding capacity (TIBC) tests, used to calculate my transferrin saturation level as described on page 243. The resulting value, 22.6 percent, is well below the 62-percent-or-higher range exhibited by men with iron overload. The other entries record the dates on which I donated blood and my serum ferritin and self-test scores. These are further discussed in the text and in Figure 20-2.

The Author's Iron Level After Donating Blood

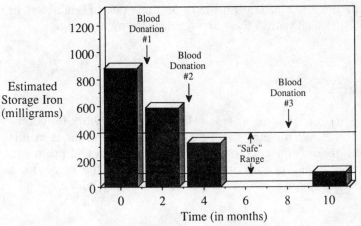

Figure 20-2. The author's iron level after donating blood. This graph shows my iron level before and after donating blood. I had serum ferritin measurements taken at each stage so that I could accurately estimate the amount of storage iron in my body. I was able to drop my iron level to within the "safe" range, 100–400 milligrams, with only two blood donations. After the second donation, I waited several months before donating again; this third donation also kept me within the safe range.

After reaching the 330-milligram level, I knew I was within the "safe" 100–400 milligram low-risk range. Thus, I waited a few months before my next donation. This third donation reduced my iron level to 110 milligrams, well within the optimal range.

Throughout my donating schedule, I felt great! I overcame my squeamishness about blood donation; just as I'd been told I would, I felt less anxiety at each subsequent session. Knowing that I was helping a number of people with my donation felt good too. The "donor's high" the experts talk about truly exists!

Did my low iron levels give me "that run-down feeling" so often mentioned in those old Geritol commercials? Not at all. I had no problem maintaining my normal furious work schedule, writing this book while holding a full-time research and faculty position. (As you can see from my diary, I had an accurate hemoglobin measurement taken to see if my low iron stores had made me anemic. The result, 14.3 grams per 100 milliliters of blood, is well within the normal range for men my age.)

Your Turn

I'm sure that the Iron Balance Health Plan will work for you as well as it has for me. As I've mentioned several times in this book, there is no guarantee that low iron levels will make you live longer, but you will have the peace of mind that comes from doing everything you can to protect your good health.

21

Answers to Common Questions About Iron Balance

I *thought iron was good for me. What has happened to change this long-standing view?*

Iron is still good for you, but *too much* iron is not.

Iron has always been a popular nutrient. This is due to cultural notions such as "iron equals strength" and the fact that the prevalence of iron deficiency in the U.S. has constantly been exaggerated. Iron seems to be a tough habit for us to break.

Now we are confronted with *new* information about iron's dark side. Scientists have uncovered the fact that iron may play an important role in the development of several diseases. It has also been discovered that an inherited form of iron overload is much more common than most doctors thought: there are more iron-overloaded men in the U.S. than iron-deficient men! Most of these findings are quite recent, and they have yet to disseminate into mainstream medicine. And a great deal more work must be done to prove "beyond a shadow of a doubt" that iron is involved in each case. But it is clear that we can never look at iron the same way again.

Is the Iron Balance Health Plan similar to chelation therapy used to remove minerals from hardened arteries?

NO! Chelation therapy is a misguided, unproven quack treatment that purports to reverse atherosclerosis by removing calcium, not iron, from plaque that deposits on artery walls. While this plaque does contain calcium, attempting to remove it with special drugs has absolutely no effect on the progress of this very complex disease of the artery wall. In addition, the treatment can be dangerous. The U.S. Food and Drug Administration has labeled chelation therapy as one of the top ten health frauds.

Iron Balance is a natural, preventive regimen that protects against excessive iron accumulation. While the effectiveness of the program in preventing several diseases has not been tested in large clinical studies, it *is* supported by a large body of scientific evidence.

Are Geritol and other iron-containing supplements actually bad for me?

Iron products are more like drugs than supplements. As such, they should only be used if recommended or prescribed by a physician in order to treat iron-deficiency anemia, or to prevent it during pregnancy. *Any drug* is potentially dangerous if used inappropriately, excessively, or, in some cases, in combination with other drugs. Iron is no different in this regard. While small doses of this drug will definitely cause no harm, chronic use can contribute to iron accumulation in several organs, sometimes leading to serious damage.

If my diet is low in iron, won't it also be low in other minerals or other important nutrients?

Dietary measures to restrict iron absorption, such as cutting down on meat and increasing the consumption of foods like wheat bran, may also decrease the amount of zinc, vitamin B12, protein, and other nutrients absorbed from your diet. However, deficiencies of these nutrients are quite rare, and as long as you're eating a balanced diet including low-fat dairy products, you'll be fine.

Can donating blood actually prevent some diseases and make me healthier?

The evidence to date suggests, but does not prove, that blood donation to remove excess iron may have health benefits. One can argue that there is a parallel to cholesterol: reduced cholesterol can result in decreased risk of heart disease for some people. Similarly, reducing iron levels may help prevent *some* diseases in *some* people, but it will take a great deal of research before we know who will benefit the most.

Can donating blood make me anemic?

Yes, if you donate too frequently. That's why there are regulations prohibiting people from donating more often than once every eight weeks. Even with this precaution, a few people will become iron-deficient, particularly younger women. If you feel excessively tired or experience shortness of breath upon exertion for several days after donating, you might have mild iron-deficiency anemia. Contact the donor center and/or your doctor and follow the recommendations in Chapter 15 for the diagnosis and treatment of this usually mild condition.

Epilogue

Iron Balance and the Next Wave in Disease Prevention

Iron Balance is control: control over the level of excess iron in your body. By following the simple rules and suggestions in the Iron Balance Health Plan, you can maintain your iron levels within the optimal range and increase your odds for a long and healthy life.

This self-control of a crucial but potentially harmful nutrient in your body fits well into tomorrow's health care environment. Largely as a result of rising costs, the individual will have to play a larger role in medicine. Self-medication with powerful drugs—properly labeled, of course—home-testing kits, and home care are part of this trend. The individual's responsibility in the area of disease prevention will become even more important than it is today. As new scientific findings are reported, you will have to choose whether or not to modify your life-style, as you have done by beginning the Iron Balance Health Plan.

As I have cautioned throughout this book, a tremendous amount of research, much of it now in progress or in the planning stages, must still be done to clarify iron's role in aging and in different diseases. Directly or indirectly, you can be part of this research. By taking commonsense measures to reduce the amount of iron, fat, and cholesterol in your body, your health and vitality will speak of the importance of both old and new preventive steps. You can be assured that the public and the medical community will take note.

As iron's good-for-you image is replaced in people's minds by a more balanced picture, I hope we see some improvements in our approach to this double-edged nutrient.

I hope that we can develop a more sensible approach to defining iron deficiency and estimating its prevalence.

I hope that the major food corporations can see the light and begin to offer whole-grain breakfast cereals, flour, and bread free of contaminating iron supplements.

I hope that there will be greater awareness of and routine screening for hemochromatosis, the inherited iron-overload disease, which threatens the health of over one million Americans. We also need warning labels for hemochromatosis victims on all foods and supplements containing added iron. If we have warning labels for the 20,000 or so phenylketonurics in this country who cannot metabolize Nutrasweet (aspartame), then why not take the same measures for the iron-overloaded?

I hope that there will be a further reduction in our intake of meat, particularly red meat, which increases our cholesterol and iron levels. The truth about iron should remove one of the last best chances of the growing meat lobby that has been trying to convince us that we cannot get enough iron without eating meat. The bottom line is that meat tastes good and can be part of a balanced, healthy diet, but not in the excessive amounts commonly consumed by Americans.

What else might we expect in the future? Medical science will surely develop new technologies for dealing with nature's oversights regarding how iron is handled in the body. We may soon have drugs to limit iron-induced damage to vital organs. Such drugs could be administered when the blockage in a coronary artery is removed and iron begins to contribute to heart muscle damage. Other drugs could be used to remove excess iron from the body, particularly when the patient cannot withstand blood removal, the best method for reducing iron levels. Similar chemicals, if proved safe, could be used as food additives to inhibit the absorption of iron from plant-based foods. Finally, we can hope that from molecular biology, the fastest growing segment of medical science, will come true miracle cures permitting errant genes to be replaced or supplemented with normal, productive ones. Inherited diseases such as hemochromatosis and inherited tendencies for such diseases as heart disease may cease to exist.

In addition to corrections in our approach to dietary iron, there will surely be many other advances to lengthen and improve the quality of our lives. But since iron appears to contribute to a process fundamental to aging itself, I wonder how effective the new measures will be in the absence of iron control. It appears to me that we must begin by removing that iron slave ring, which holds our health hostage, from around our necks.

Armed with the Iron Balance Health Plan, you can be part of this future now.

References

Chapter 1. Our One-Sided View of Iron

1. *Oxford English Dictionary*. Oxford: Oxford University Press, 1986.
2. Plinius, G., III. *The Historie of the World*, Book 34, Chapter IV. (Holland translation.) London: Adam Islip, 1601.
3. Fairbanks, V. F.; Fahey, J. L.; Beutler, E. *Clinical Disorders of Iron Metabolism*. New York: Grune & Stratton, 1971; chapter 1.
4. Scala, J. *Making the Vitamin Connection*. New York: Harper & Row, 1985; chapter 8.
5. Guggenheim, K. Y. *Nutrition and Nutritional Diseases*. Lexington, MA: Collamore Press, 1981; chapter 13.
6. Fowler, W. M. "Chlorosis—An Obituary." *Ann. Med. Hist.* 1936, 8, 168–177.
7. Major, R. H. *Classic Descriptions of Disease*. Springfield, IL: Charles C. Thomas, 1932; pp. 444–447.
8. Crosby, W. H. "Whatever Became of Chlorosis?" *Journal of the American Medical Association*, 1987, 257, 2799–2800.

Chapter 2. Iron in Your Body: Freeways and Dead Ends

1. National Research Council. *Iron*. Baltimore: University Park Press, 1979; chapters 2–4.
2. Bothwell, T. H.; Charlton, R. W.; Cook, J. D.; Finch, C. A. *Iron Metabolism In Man*. Oxford: Blackwell Scientific Publications, 1979.
3. Hallberg, L. In *Nutrition Reviews' Present Knowledge in Nutrition*. Washington, D.C.: The Nutrition Foundation, 1984; chapter 32.

4. Wheby, M. S. In *Fundamentals of Clinical Hematology*, Thorup, O. A., ed., 5th Edition. Philadelphia: Saunders, 1987; chapter 10.

5. Widdowson, E. M. In *Nutrition in the 20th Century*, Winick, M., ed. New York: John Wiley & Sons, 1984; chapter 1.

6. Marx, J. J. M. "Normal Iron Absorption and Decreased Red Cell Iron Uptake in the Aged." *Blood* 1979, 53, 204–211.

7. Casale, G.; Bonora, C.; Migliavacca, A.; Zurita, I.; de Nicola, P. "Serum Ferritin and Ageing." *Age and Ageing* 1981, 10, 119–122.

8. Cook, J. D. "Adaptation in Iron Metabolism." *American Journal of Clinical Nutrition* 1990, 51, 301–308.

9. Cook, J. D.; Finch, C. A.; Smith, N. J. "Evaluation of the Iron Status of a Population." *Blood* 1976, 48, 449–455.

10. Leggett, B. A.; Brown, N. N.; Bryant, S. J.; Duplock, L.; Powell, L. W.; Halliday, J. W. "Factors Affecting the Concentrations of Ferritin in Serum in a Healthy Australian Population." *Clinical Chemistry* 1990, 36, 1350–1355.

11. Theil, E. C. "Ferritin: Structure, Gene Regulation, and Cellular Function in Animals, Plants, and Microorganisms." *Annual Review of Biochemistry*, 1987, 56, 289–315.

12. Crichton, R. R. "Iron Uptake and Utilization by Mammalian Cells: II. Intracellular Iron Utilization." *Trends in Biochemical Science* 1984, 9, 283–286.

13. Halliwell, B.; Gutteridge, J. M. C. "Iron and Free Radical Reactions: Two Aspects of Antioxidant Protection." *Trends in Biochemical Science*, September 1989, 372–375.

14. Cross, C. E., et al. "Oxygen Radicals and Human Disease." *Ann. Int. Med.* 1987, 107, 526–545.

Chapter 3. The Geritol Scam

1. *Federal Trade Commission Decisions* 1965, 68, 481–555; 1968, 74, 1632–1641; 1972, 81, 238–245.

2. Gold, P. *Advertising, Politics, and American Culture: From Salesmanship to Therapy*. New York: Paragon House, 1987; p. 164.

3. Cox, E. F.; Fellmeth, R. C.; Schulz, J. E. *The Nader Report on*

the Federal Trade Commission. New York: Richard W. Baron, 1969.

4. *New York Times,* July 5, 1969; December 4, 1969; April 21, 1970; January 23, 1973; January 14, 1976.

5. *Wall Street Journal,* April 21, 1970; January 23, 1973; January 14, 1976.

6. Herbert, V.; Barrett, S. *Vitamins and Health Foods: The Great American Hustle.* Philadelphia: George F. Stickley Company, 1981; chapter 12.

Chapter 4. Politics and the Mismeasuring of Anemia

1. Kotz, N. *Let Them Eat Promises: The Politics of Hunger in America.* Englewood Cliffs, NJ: Prentice-Hall, 1969.

2. Schlesinger, A. M. *Robert Kennedy and His Times.* Boston: Houghton Mifflin, 1978; pp. 794–800.

3. Anson, R. S. *McGovern: A Biography.* New York: Holt, Rinehart and Winston, 1972; chapter 10.

4. *Ten State Nutrition Survey 1968–1970. IV. Biochemical Data.* DHEW publication no. (HSM) 72-8132. Atlanta: US Dept. of Health, Education, and Welfare, Centers For Disease Control, 1972.

5. Crosby, W. H. "Serum Ferritin and Iron Enrichment." *Journal of the American Medical Association,* 1974, 290, 1435–1436.

6. Beaton, G. H. "Epidemiology of Iron Deficiency." In *Iron in Biochemistry and Medicine,* Jacobs, A.; Worwood, M., eds. London: Academic Press, 1974; chapter 13.

7. U.S. Senate Select Committee on Nutrition and Human Needs. *Nutrition and Health with an Evaluation of Nutritional Surveillance in the U.S.* Washington, D.C.: U.S. Government Printing Office, 1975.

8. Expert Scientific Working Group. "Summary of a Report on Assessment of the Iron Nutritional Status of the United States Population." *American Journal of Clinical Nutrition,* 1985, 42, 1318–1330.

9. Dallman, P. R. "Prevalence and Causes of Anemia in the

United States, 1976–1980." *American Journal of Clinical Nutrition*, 1984, 39, 437–445.

10. Food and Nutrition Board, Commission on Life Sciences, National Research Council. *What Is America Eating?* Washington, D.C.: National Academy Press, 1986.

11. Herbert, V. "Recommended Dietary Intakes (RDI) of Iron in Humans." *American Journal of Clinical Nutrition*, 1987, 45, 679–86.

Chapter 5. Anemia Today: Overdiagnosed and Overtreated

1. Podell, R. *Doctor, Why Am I So Tired?* New York: Pharos Books, 1988.

2. Waller, D. G.; Smith, A. G. "Attitudes to Prescribing Iron Supplements in General Practice." *British Medical Journal* 1987, 294, 94–96.

3. Oppenheim, M. "The Five Most Overdiagnosed Diseases." *Cosmopolitan*, May 1984, 152.

4. Elwood, P. C. "The Enrichment Debate." *Nutrition Today* July/August 1977, 18–24.

5. Finch, C. A.; Cook, J. D. "Iron Deficiency." *American Journal of Clinical Nutrition*, 1984, 39, 471–477.

6. Dallman, P. R. "Iron Deficiency and the Immune Response." *American Journal of Clinical Nutrition*, 1987, 46, 329–334.

7. Wheby, M. S. In *Fundamentals of Clinical Hematology*, Thorup, O. A., ed., 5th Edition. Philadelphia: Saunders, 1987; chapter 10.

Chapter 6. Fortification Follies

1. Hamilton, E. M. N.; Whitney, E. N. *Nutrition: Concepts and Controversies*. St. Paul: West Publishing, 1982; chapters 3, 10, and 11.

2. Vetter, J. L., ed. *Adding Nutrients to Foods: Where Do We Go From Here?* St. Paul: American Association of Cereal Chemists, 1982.

3. Hunter, B. T. "Proposed Sharp Increase in Addition of Iron to Wheat Flour and Bread." *Consumer Bulletin* November 1972, 29–31.

4. *Federal Register* October 15, 1973 (Vol. 38, No. 198), 28558; February 11, 1974 (Vol. 39, No. 29), 5188; October 19, 1976 (Vol. 41, No. 203), 46156; August 29, 1978 (Vol. 43, No. 168), 38575; March 16, 1979 (Vol. 44, No. 53), 16005; October 19, 1979 (Vol. 44, No. 204), 60313.

5. Crosby, W. H. "Yin, Yang and Iron." *Nutrition Today* July/August 1986, 14–16.

6. Elwood, P. C. "The Enrichment Debate." *Nutrition Today* July/August 1977, 18–24.

7. Crosby, W. H. "Serum Ferritin and Iron Enrichment." *New England Journal of Medicine* 1974, 290, 1435–1436.

8. Krikker, M. A. "Body Iron Stores and the Risk of Cancer." *New England Journal of Medicine,* 1989, 320, 1012–1013.

9. Anonymous. *Business Week* March 29, 1976, 36.

10. White, H. S. "Freedom of Choice." *Journal of Nutrition Education,* 1978, 10 (October–December), 150–151.

11. Patner, A. "Dr. Demopoulos Sells a 'Fountain of Youth' to Rich and Famous." *Wall Street Journal,* November 8, 1989; p. A1, A12.

12. Hausman, P. *The Right Dose: How to Take Vitamins and Minerals Safely.* New York: Ballantine Books, 1987; chapter 1.

13. American Pharmaceutical Association. *Handbook of Nonprescription Drugs.* Washington, D.C.: American Pharmaceutical Association, 1990 (9th edition).

14. Anonymous. *Advertising Age* 1989, 60 (Sept. 27), 88–94.

15. Maxwell, J. C. "Cereal Market Up, No. 1 Kellogg Down." *Advertising Age* 1989, 60 (Sept. 25), 27.

16. Harvard Business School Case Study #9-582-114, "Total Cereal" (1982).

17. General Mills, Minneapolis, Minnesota.

18. Belasco, W. J. *Appetite for Change: How the Counterculture Took On the Food Industry.* New York: Pantheon Books, 1989; p. 218.

19. Crosby, W. H. "The Safety of Iron-Fortified Food." *Journal of the American Medical Association,* 1978, 239, 2026–2027.

20. Olsson, K. S.; Heedman, P. A.; Staugard, F. "Preclinical Hemochromatosis in a Population on a High-Iron-Fortified

Diet." *Journal of the American Medical Association*, 1978, 239, 1999–2000.

21. *Ironic Blood* January/February 1990, Vol. 10, No. 1. North Palm Beach, FL: Iron Overload Disease Association.

Chapter 7. Hereditary Iron-Overload Disease: A Hidden Killer

1. Fairbanks, V. F.; Fahey, J. L.; Beutler, E. *Clinical Disorders of Iron Metabolism*. New York: Grune & Stratton, 1971; chapter 1.

2. MacDonald, R. A. *Hemochromatosis and Hemosiderosis*. Springfield, IL: Charles C. Thomas, 1964.

3. Bothwell, T. H.; Charlton, R. W.; Cook, J. D.; Finch, C. A. *Iron Metabolism in Man*. Oxford: Blackwell Scientific Publications, 1979.

4. Edwards, C. Q.; Griffen, L. M.; Goldgar, D.; Drummond, C.; Skolnick, M. H.; Kushner, J. P. "Prevalence of Hemochromatosis Among 11,065 Presumably Healthy Blood Donors." *New England Journal of Medicine*, 1988, 318, 1355–1362.

5. Beaudet, A. L.; Scriver, C. R.; Sly, W. S.; Valle, D. "Genetics and Biochemistry of Variant Human Phenotypes." In *The Metabolic Basis of Inherited Disease*, Scriver, C. R., et al., eds. New York: McGraw-Hill, 1989; chapter 1.

6. *Ironic Blood* September/October 1985, Vol. 5, No. 4; September/October 1988, Vol. 8, No. 5; November/December 1989, Vol. 9, No. 6; March/April 1990, Vol. 10, No. 2. Iron Overload Diseases Association, West Palm Beach, Florida.

7. Bothwell, T. H.; Charlton, R. W.; Motulsky, A. G. "Hemochromatosis." In *The Metabolic Basis of Inherited Disease*, Scriver, C. R., et al., eds. New York:, McGraw-Hill, 1989; chapter 55.

8. Summers, K. M.; Halliday, J. W.; Powell, L. W. "Identification of Homozygous Hemochromatosis Subjects by Measurement of Hepatic Iron Index." *Hepatology* 1990, 12, 20–25.

9. Niederau, C.; Fischer, R.; Sonnenberg, A.; Stremmel, W.;

Trampisch, H. J.; Strohmeyer, G. "Survival and Causes of Death in Cirrhotic and in Noncirrhotic Patients with Primary Hemochromatosis." *New England Journal of Medicine*, 1985, 313, 1256–1263.

10. Crawford, R. "My Body Was Rusting Away." *Good Housekeeping*, November 1980, pp. 122–126.
11. Crosby, W. H. "Hemochromatosis: The Missed Diagnosis." *Arch. Intern. Med.* 1986, 146, 1209–1210.
12. "Case Records of the Massachusetts General Hospital." *New England Journal of Medicine*, 1983, 308, 1521–1529.

Chapter 8. Other Causes of Iron Overload

1. MacDonald, R. A. *Hemochromatosis and Hemosiderosis*. Springfield, IL: Charles C. Thomas, 1964.
2. Bothwell, T. H.; Charlton, R. W.; Cook, J. D.; Finch, C. A. *Iron Metabolism in Man*. Oxford: Blackwell Scientific Publications, 1979.
3. Campbell, D. *In the Heart of Bantuland*. New York: Negro Universities Press, 1969.
4. Murphy, E. J. *The Bantu Civilization of Southern Africa*. New York: Thomas Y. Crowell Company, 1974.
5. Anonymous. "Case Records of the Massachusetts General Hospital." *New England Journal of Medicine*, 1952, 247, 992–995.
6. Green, P.; Eviatar, J. M.; Sirota, P.; Avidor, I. "Secondary Hemochromatosis Due to Prolonged Iron Ingestion." *Israel Journal of Medicical Sciences* 1989, 25, 199–201.
7. Johnson, B. F. "Hemochromatosis Resulting From Prolonged Oral Iron Therapy." *New England Journal of Medicine* 1968, 278, 1100–1101.
8. Turnberg, L. A. "Excessive Oral Iron Therapy Causing Hemochromatosis." *British Medical Journal* 1965, 1, 1360.
9. Herbert, V. "Recommended Dietary Intakes (RDI) of Iron in Humans." *American Journal of Clinical Nutrition*, 1987, 45, 679–686.
10. Sas, F.; Nemesanszky, E.; Brauer, H.; Scheffer, K. *"Auch*

Dreiwertiges Eisen Wird Resorbiert." *Munch. med. Wochenschr.* 1984, 126, 1063–1068.

11. Sas, F.; Nemesanszky, E.; Brauer, H.; Scheffer, K. "On the Therapeutic Effects of Trivalent and Divalent Iron in Iron Deficiency Anemia." *Arzneim.-Forsch.* 1984, 34, 1575–1579.

Chapter 9. Iron and Heart Disease

1. *World Health Statistics Annual.* World Health Organization, Geneva, 1981–1988.
2. Soldo, B. J.; Manton, K. G. "Demography: Characteristics and Implications of an Aging Population." In *Geriatric Medicine*, Rowe, J. W., and Besdine, R. W., eds. Boston: Little, Brown, 1988, pp. 12–22.
3. Wingard, D. L. "The Sex Differential in Morbidity, Mortality, and Lifestyle." *Annual Review of Public Health* 1984, 5, 433–458.
4. Brody, J. E. "Countering the Myth That Women Have Little to Fear From Heart Disease." *New York Times*, February 2, 1989, p. B7.
5. Braunwald, E., ed. *Heart Disease: A Textbook of Cardiovascular Medicine.* Philadelphia: W.B. Saunders, 1988; chapter 36.
6. Gordon, T.; Kannel, W. B.; Hjortland, M. C.; McNamara, P. M. "Menopause and Risk of Cardiovascular Disease: The Framingham Study." *Ann. Intern. Med.* 1976, 85, 447–452.
7. Sullivan, J. L. "The Iron Paradigm of Ischemic Heart Disease." *American Heart Journal* 1989, 117, 1177–1188.
8. Fraser, G. E. "Determinants of Ischemic Heart Disease in Seventh-Day Adventists: A Review." *American Journal of Clinical Nutrition* 1988, 48, 833–836.
9. Sullivan, J. L. "Vegetarianism, Ischemic Heart Disease, and Iron." *American Journal of Clinical Nutrition* 1983, 37, 882–883.
10. Lauffer, R. B. "Iron Stores and the International Variation in Mortality From Coronary Artery Disease." *Medical Hypotheses* 1991, 35, 96–102.
11. Ambrosio, G.; Zweier, J. L.; Jacobus, W. E.; Weisfeldt, M. L.; Flaherty, J. T. "Improvement of Postischemic Myocardial

Dysfunction and Metabolism Induced by Administration of Deferoxamine At the Time of Reflow: The Role of Iron in the Pathogenesis of Reperfusion Injury." *Circulation* 1987, 76, 906–915.

12. McCord, J. M. "Is Iron Sufficiency a Risk Factor in Ischemic Heart Disease?" *Circulation* 1991, 83, 1112–1114.

13. Davies, S. W.; Ranjadayalan, K.; Wickens, D. G.; Dormandy, T. L.; Timmis, A. D. "Lipid Peroxidation Associated with Successful Thrombolysis." *Lancet* 1990, 335, 741–743.

14. Steinberg, D.; Parthasarathy, S.; Carew, T. E.; Khoo, J. C.; Witztum, J. L. "Beyond Cholesterol: Modifications of Low-Density Lipoprotein That Increase Its Atherogenicity." *New England Journal of Medicine*, 1989, 320, 915–924.

15. Kuzuya, M.; Naito, M.; Yamada, K.; Funaki, C.; Hayashi, T.; Asai, K.; Kuzuya, F. "Involvement of Intracellular Iron in the Toxicity of Oxidized Low Density Lipoprotein to Cultured Endothelial Cells." *Biochemistry International* 1990, 22, 567–573.

16. Koten, J.; McWethy, V. L. "Do As We Do: Our Survey Shows Cardiologists Take Their Own Advice to Heart." *Wall Street Journal*, May 11, 1990; p. R27.

17. Lauffer, R. B. "Exercise, Fitness, and Mortality." *Journal of the American Medical Association*, 1990, 263, 2047.

18. Lauffer, R. B. "Exercise as Prevention: Do the Health Benefits Derive in Part From Lower Iron Levels?" *Medical Hypotheses 1991, 35, 103–107.*

19. Lauffer, R. B. "Iron Depletion and Coronary Disease." *American Heart Journal* 1990, 119, 1448.

Chapter 10. Iron and Brain Disorders

1. Krause, G. S.; White, B. C.; Aust, S. D.; Nayini, N. R.; Kumar, K. "Brain Cell Death Following Ischemia and Reperfusion: A Proposed Biochemical Sequence." *Critical Care Medicine* 1988, 16, 714–726.

2. Patt, A.; Horesh, I. R.; Berger, E. M.; Harken, A. H.; Repine, J. E. "Iron Depletion or Chelation Reduces Ischemia/Reper-

fusion-Induced Edema in Gerbil Brains." *Journal of Pediatric Surgery*, 1990, 25, 224–228.

3. Marsden, D. D. "Parkinson's Disease." *Lancet*, 1990, 335, 948–952.

4. Youdim, M. B. H.; Ben-Shachar, D.; Riederer, P. "Is Parkinson's Disease a Progressive Siderosis of Substantia Nigra Resulting in Iron and Melanin Induced Neurodegeneration?" *Acta Neurol. Scand.* 1989, 126, 47–54.

5. Birchall, J. D.; Chappell, J. S. "Aluminum, Chemical Physiology, and Alzheimer's Disease." *Lancet* 1988 (October 29), pp. 1008–1010.

6. Martyn, C. N.; Barker, D. J. P.; Osmond, C.; Harris, E. C.; Edwardson, J. A.; Lacey, R. F. "Geographical Relation Between Alzheimer's Disease and Aluminum in Drinking Water." *Lancet* 1989, i, 59–62.

7. Farrar, G.; Altmann, P.; Welch, S., et al. "Defective Gallium-Transferrin Binding in Alzheimer Disease and Down Syndrome: Possible Mechanism for Accumulation of Aluminum in Brain." *Lancet* 1990, 335, 747–750.

8. McLachlan, D. R. C.; Dalton, A. J.; Kruck, T. P. A.; Bell, M. Y.; Smith, W. L.; Kalow, W.; Andrews, D. F. "Intramuscular Desferrioxamine in Patients With Alzheimer's Disease." *Lancet* 1991, 337 (June 1), 1304–1308.

Chapter 11. Iron and Cancer

1. a. Ames, B. N. Lecture, Massachusetts Institute of Technology, May 15, 1990. b. Ames, B. N. "Dietary Carcinogens and Anticarcinogens." *Science* 1983, 221, 1256–1264. c. Cross, C. E.; Halliwell, B.; Borish, E. T.; Pryor, W. A.; Ames, B. N.; Saul, R. L.; McCord, J. M.; Harman, D. "Oxygen Radicals and Human Disease." *Ann. Intern. Med.* 1987, 107, 526–545.

2. Crosby, W. H. "Yin, Yang and Iron." *Nutrition Today* 1986, July/August, 14–16.

3. Krikker, M. A. "Body Iron Stores and the Risk of Cancer." *New England Journal of Medicine*, 1989, 320, 1012–1013.

4. Hann, H. L.; Stahlhut, M. W.; Blumberg, B. S. "Iron Nutrition and Tumor Growth: Decreased Tumor Growth in Iron-Deficient Mice." *Cancer Research* 1988, 48, 4168–4170.

5. Nelson, R. L.; Yoo, S. J.; Tanure, J. C.; Andrianopoulos, G.; Misumi, A. "The Effect of Iron on Experimental Colorectal Carcinogenesis." *Anticancer Research* 1989, 9, 1477–1482.

6. Weinberg, E. D. "Iron Withholding: A Defense Against Infection and Neoplasia." *Physiol. Rev.* 1984, 64, 65–102.

7. Stevens, R. G.; Jones, D. Y.; Micozzi, M. S.; Taylor, P. R. "Body Iron Stores and the Risk of Cancer." *New England Journal of Medicine*, 1988, 319, 1047–1052.

8. Stevens, R. G.; Kuvibidila, S.; Kapps, M.; Friedlaender, J.; Blumberg, B. S. "Iron-binding Proteins, Hepatitis B Virus, and Mortality in the Solomon Islands." *American Journal of Epidemiology*, 1983, 118, 550–561.

9. Stevens, R. G.; Beasley, R. P.; Blumberg, B. S. "Iron-binding Proteins and Risk of Cancer in Taiwan." *Journal of the National Cancer Institute* 1986, 76, 605–610.

10. Selby, J. V.; Friedman, G. D. "Epidemiologic Evidence of an Association Between Body Iron Stores and Risk of Cancer." *International Journal of Cancer* 1988, 41, 677–682.

11. Cohen, L. A. "Diet and Cancer." *Scientific American* 1987, 257 (November), 42–48.

12. MacLennan, R.; Jensen, O. M.; Mosbech, J.; Vuori, H. "Diet, Transit Time, Stool Weight, and Colon Cancer in Two Scandinavian Populations." *American Journal of Clinical Nutrition*, 1978, 31, S239–S242.

13. Jensen, O. M.; MacLennan, R. "Dietary Factors and Colorectal Cancer in Scandinavia." *Israel Journal of Medical Science* 1979, 15, 329–334.

14. MacLennan, R.; Jensen, O. M. "Dietary Fibre, Transit-Time, Faecal Bacteria, Steroids, and Colon Cancer in Two Scandinavian Populations." *Lancet* 1977, 2 (8031), 207–211.

15. Glober, G. A.; Kamiyama, S.; Nomura, A.; Shimada, A.; Abba, B. C. "Bowel Transit-Time and Stool Weight in Populations with Different Colon-Cancer Risks." *Lancet* 1977, 2 (8029), 110–111.

16. Graf, E.; Eaton, J. W. "Dietary Suppression of Colonic Cancer: Fiber or Phytate?" *Cancer* 1985, 56, 717–718.

17. Graf, E.; Empson, K. L.; Eaton, J. W. "Phytic Acid: A Natural Antioxidant." *Journal of Biological Chemistry* 1987, 262, 11647–11650.
18. Irving, D.; Drasar, B. S. "Fibre and Cancer of the Colon." *British Journal of Cancer*, 1973, 28, 462–463.

Chapter 12. Iron and Aging

1. Harman, D. "Free Radical Theory of Aging: Role of Free Radicals in the Origination and Evolution of Life, Aging, and Disease Processes." In *Free Radicals, Aging, and Degenerative Diseases*, Johnson, J. E.; Walford, R.; Harman, D.; Miquel, J., eds. Alan R. Liss, Inc., New York, 1986; pp. 3–50.
2. Cross, C. E.; Halliwell, B.; Borish, E. T.; Pryor, W. A.; Ames, B. N.; Saul, R. L.; McCord, J. M.; Harman, D. "Oxygen Radicals and Human Disease." *Ann. Intern. Med.* 1987, 107, 526–545.
3. Halliwell, B.; Gutteridge, J. M. C. *Free Radicals in Biology and Medicine.* Oxford: Clarendon Press, 1985.
4. Katz, M. L.; Robison, W. G. "Nutritional Influences on Autoxidation, Lipofuscin Accumulation, and Aging." In *Free Radicals, Aging, and Degenerative Diseases*, Johnson, J. E., Walford, R., Harman, D., Miquel, J., eds. New York: Alan. R. Liss, 1986; pp. 221–262.
5. Marzabadi, M. R.; Sohal, R. S.; Brunk, U. T. "Effect of Ferric Iron and Desferrioxamine on Lipofuscin Accumulation in Cultured Rat Heart Myocytes." *Mech. Ageing Devel.* 1988, 46, 145–157.
6. Merry, P.; Kidd, B.; Blake, D. "Modification of Rheumatic Symptoms by Diet and Drugs." *Proc. Nutr. Soc.* 1989, 48, 363–369.
7. Pearson, D.; Shaw, S. *Life Extension.* New York: Warner Books, 1982.

Chapter 13. The Iron-Depletion Hypothesis: Less Is Best

1. Martin, W. "Do We Get Too Much Iron?" *Medical Hypotheses* 1984, 14, 131–133.
2. Stevens, R. G.; Kalkwarf, D. R. "Iron, Radiation, and Cancer." *Environmental Health Perspectives* 1990, 87, 291–300.
3. Sullivan, J. L. "The Iron Paradigm of Ischemic Heart Disease." *American Heart Journal* 1989, 117, 1177–1188.
4. Weinberg, R. J.; Ell, S. R.; Weinberg, E. D. "Blood-Letting, Iron Homeostasis, and Human Health." *Medical Hypotheses* 1986, 21, 441–443.
5. Weinberg, E. D. "Iron Withholding: A Defense Against Infection and Neoplasia." *Physiological Reviews* 1984, 64, 65–102.
6. Weinberg, E. D. "Cellular Iron Metabolism in Health and Disease." *Drug Metabolism Reviews* 1990, 22, 531–579.
7. Ell, S. R. "Iron in Two Seventeenth-Century Plague Epidemics." *Journal of Interdisciplinary History* 1985 (Winter), 15, 445–457.

Chapter 15. Iron Balance for Women and Children

1. Weideger, P. *Menstruation and Menopause*. New York: Alfred Knopf, 1976; chapters 1 and 4.
2. Frassinelli-Gunderson, E. P.; Margen, S.; Brown, J. R. "Iron Stores in Users of Oral Contraceptive Agents." *American Journal of Clinical Nutrition*, 1985, 41, 703–712.
3. Expert Scientific Working Group. "Summary of a Report on Assessment of the Iron Nutritional Status of the United States Population." *American Journal of Clinical Nutrition*, 1985, 42, 1318–1330.
4. Crosby, W. H. "The Rationale for Treating Iron Deficiency Anemia." *Arch. Intern. Med.* 1984, 144, 471–472.
5. Crosby, W. H. "Overtreating the Deficiency Anemias." *Arch. Intern. Med.* 1986, 146, 779.
6. Herbert, V. "Recommended Dietary Intakes (RDI) of Iron

in Humans." *American Journal of Clinical Nutrition*, 1987, 45, 679–686.

7. Cunningham, F. G.; MacDonald, P. C.; Gant, N. F. *Williams Obstetrics* (Eighteenth Edition). Norwalk, CT: Appleton & Lange, 1989; chapters 7 and 14.

8. Hibbard, B. M. "Iron and Folate Supplements During Pregnancy: Supplementation Is Valuable Only in Selected Patients." *British Medical Journal*, 1988, 297, 1324, 1326.

9. Jovanovic-Peterson, L. "Guest Editorial: What Is So Bad About a Prolonged Pregnancy?" *Journal of the American College of Nutrition* 1991, 10, 1–2.

10. Hemminki, E.; Rimpela, U. "A Randomized Comparison of Routine Versus Selective Iron Supplementation During Pregnancy." *Journal of the American College of Nutrition* 1991, 10, 3–10.

11. Sullivan, J. L. "Iron, Plasma Antioxidants, and the 'Oxygen Radical Disease of Prematurity'." *Amer. J. Dis. Child.* 1988, 142, 1341–1344.

12. Sullivan, J. L. "Bronchopulmonary Dysplasia, Undernutrition, and Iron." *Amer. Rev. Resp. Dis.* 1989, 139, 850.

13. Taylor, J. A.; Bergman, A. B. "Iron-Fortified Formulas: Pediatricians' Prescribing Practices." *Clinical Pediatrics* 1989, 28, 73–75.

14. Dallman, P. R. "Upper Limits of Iron in Infant Formulas." *Journal of Nutrition*, 1989, 119, 1852–1855.

15. Dagnelie, P. C.; van Staveren, W. A.; Vergote, F.; Dingjan, P. G.; van den Berg, H.; Hautvast, J. G. "Increased Risk of Vitamin B-12 and Iron Deficiency in Infants on Macrobiotic Diets." *Amer. J. Clin. Nutr.* 1989, 50, 818–824.

Chapter 16. Optimal Health Through Optimal Nutrition: The Low-Fat, Low-Iron Life-style

1. Ornish, D. *Dr. Dean Ornish's Program for Reversing Heart Disease.* New York: Random House, 1990.

2. Brody, J. E. *Jane Brody's Good Food Book.* New York: Bantam Books, 1987; chapter 1.

3. Farb, P.; Armelagos, G. *Consuming Passions: The Anthropology of Eating.* Boston: Houghton Mifflin, 1980.

4. Garn, S. M.; Leonard, W. R. "What Did Our Ancestors Eat?" *Nutrition Reviews* 1989, 47, 337–345.

5. Lee, R. B.; deVore, I., eds. *Kalahari Hunter-Gatherers*. Cambridge, MA: Harvard University Press, 1976.

6. Brody, J. E. "Huge Study of Diet Indicts Fat and Meat." *New York Times*, May 8, 1990; p. C1, C14.

7. American Dietetic Association. "Position of the American Dietetic Association on Vegetarian Diets—Technical Support Paper." *ADA Reports* 1988, 88, 352–355.

8. Burros, M. "Rethink Four Food Groups, Doctors Tell U.S." *New York Times*, April 10, 1991; pp. C1, C4.

9. Cook, J. D. "Adaptation in Iron Metabolism." *American Journal of Clinical Nutrition*, 1990, 51, 301–308.

10. Leggett, B. A.; Brown, N. N.; Bryant, S. J.; Duplock, L.; Powell, L. W.; Halliday, J. W. "Factors Affecting the Concentrations of Ferritin in Serum in a Healthy Australian Population." *Clinical Chemistry* 1990, 36, 1350–1355.

11. Widdowson, E. M.; McCance, R. A. "Iron Exchanges of Adults on White and Brown Bread." *Lancet* 1942, 1, 588–591.

12. Graf. E.; Eaton, J. W. "Dietary Suppression of Colonic Cancer: Fiber or Phytate?" *Cancer* 1985, 56, 717–718.

13. Graf. E.; Eaton, J. W. "Antioxidant Functions of Phytic Acid." *Free Radical Biology and Medicine* 1990, 8, 61–69.

14. Irving, D.; Drasar, B. S. "Fibre and Cancer of the Colon." *British Journal of Cancer* 1973, 28, 462–463.

15. McKeown-Eyssen, G. E.; Bright-See, E. "Dietary Factors in Colon Cancer: International Relationships." *Nutrition and Cancer* 1984, 6, 160–170.

16. Lappé, F. M. *Diet for a Small Planet*. New York: Ballantine, 1975.

17. *New York Times*, March 21, 1990; July 18, 1990.

Chapter 17. The Iron Balance Diet

1. Pennington, J. A. T. *Food Values of Portions Commonly Used*, 15th Edition. New York: Harper & Row, 1989.

2. Benson, J. S. [Editorial.] *New York Times*, November 1, 1990.

3. Vartabedian, R. E.; Matthews, K. *Nutripoints.* New York: Harper & Row, 1990.

4. Ramirez, A. *New York Times,* March 13, 1991; pp. A1, A9.

5. Graf. E.; Eaton, J. W. "Dietary Suppression of Colonic Cancer: Fiber or Phytate?" *Cancer* 1985, 56, 717–718.

6. Graf. E.; Eaton, J. W. "Antioxidant Functions of Phytic Acid." *Free Radical Biology and Medicine* 1990, 8, 61–69.

7. *Food Consumption Statistics 1976–1985.* Organization for Economic Cooperation and Development, Paris, 1988.

8. Englyst, H. N.; Bingham, S. A.; Wiggins, H. S., et al. "Nonstarch Polysaccharide Consumption in Four Scandinavian Populations." *Nutrition and Cancer* 1982, 4, 50–60.

9. Nicol, G. *Finland.* London: B. T. Batsford, 1975; chapter 8.

10. Harland, B. F.; Harland, J. "Fermentive Reduction of Phytate in Rye, Wheat, and Whole Wheat Breads." *Cereal Chemistry* 1980, 57, 226–229.

11. Harland, B. F.; Prosky, L. "Development of Dietary Fiber Values for Foods." *Cereal Foods World* 1979, 24, 387–394.

12. Chapman, R. W.; Morgan, M. Y.; Bell, R.; Sherlock, S. "Hepatic Iron Uptake in Alcoholic Liver Disease." *Gastroenterology* 1983, 84, 143–147.

13. Chapman, R. W.; Morgan, M. Y.; Laulicht, M.; Hoffbrand, A. V.; Sherlock, S. "Hepatic Iron Stores and Markers of Iron Overload in Alcoholics and Patients with Idiopathic Hemochromatosis." *Digestive Diseases and Sciences* 1982, 27, 909–916.

14. Friedman, I. M.; Kraemer, H. C.; Mendoza, F. S.; Hammer, L. D. "Elevated Serum Iron Concentration in Adolescent Alcohol Users." *American Journal of Diseases of Children* 1988, 142, 156–159.

15. Nordmann, R.; Ribiere, C.; Rouach, H. "Ethanol-Induced Lipid Peroxidation and Oxidative Stress in Extrahepatic Tissues." *Alcohol & Alcoholism* 1990, 25, 231–237.

16. Rouach, H.; Houze, P.; Orfanelli, M.-T.; Gentil, M.; Bourdon, R.; Nordmann, R. "Effect of Acute Ethanol Administration on the Subcellular Distribution of Iron in Rat Liver and Cerebellum." *Biochemical Pharmacology* 1990, 39, 1095–1100.

17. Cederbaum, A. I. "Oxygen Radical Generation by Micro-

somes: Role of Iron and Implications for Alcohol Metabolism and Toxicity." *Free Radical Biology and Medicine* 1989, 7, 559–567.

18. Hilts, P. J. "U.S. Dietary Guide Sets Fat and Alcohol Limits." *New York Times*, November 6, 1990.

19. Olson, J. A.; Hodges, R. E. "Recommended Dietary Intakes (RDI) of Vitamin C in Humans." *American Journal of Clinical Nutrition*, 1987, 45, 693–703.

20. Nienhuis, A. W. "Vitamin C and Iron." *New England Journal of Medicine*, 1981, 304, 170–171.

21. McLaran, C. J.; Bett, J. H. N.; Nye, J. A.; Halliday, J. W. "Congestive Cardiomyopathy and Haemochromatosis—Rapid Progression Possibly Accelerated by Excessive Ingestion of Ascorbic Acid." *Aust. N.Z. J. Med.* 1982, 12, 187–188.

22. Marshall, E. "Academy Sued on 'Plagiarized' Diet Report." *Science* 1990 (March 2), 247, 1022.

23. Hallberg, L. In *Nutrition Reviews' Present Knowledge in Nutrition*. Washington, D.C.: The Nutrition Foundation, 1984; chapter 32.

24. Brune, M.; Rossander, L.; Hallberg, L. "Iron Absorption and Phenolic Compounds: Importance of Different Phenolic Structures." *European Journal of Clinical Nutrition*, 1989, 43, 547–558.

25. Morck, T. A.; Lynch, S. R.; Cook, J. D. "Inhibition of Food Iron Absorption by Coffee." *American Journal of Clinical Nutrition*, 1983, 37, 416–420.

26. Brody, J. E. *New York Times* March 14, 1991; p. B8.

27. Moore, C. V. "Iron Nutrition and Requirements." *Ser. Haematol.* 1965, 6, 1–14.

28. Brody, J. E. *Jane Brody's Good Food Book*. New York: Bantam Books, 1987.

29. Grundy, S.; Winston, M. *The American Heart Association Low-Fat, Low-Cholesterol Cookbook*. New York: Times Books, 1989.

30. Fisher, M. C.; Lachance, P. A. "Nutrition Evaluation of Published Weight-Reducing Diets." *Journal of the American Dietetic Association*, 1985, 85, 450–454.

31. Berger, S. M. *Dr. Berger's Immune Power Diet*. New York: New American Library, 1985.

32. Cooper, K. H. *Controlling Cholesterol*. New York: Bantam Books, 1988.
33. Katahn, M. *The T-Factor Diet*. New York: W. W. Norton & Co., 1989.

Chapter 18. Donating Blood to Remove Excess Iron

1. Burnum, J. F. "Medical Vampires." *New England Journal of Medicine* 1986, 314, 1250–1251.
2. Garrison, F. H. *An Introduction to the History of Medicine*. Philadelphia: W.B. Saunders Company, 1924.
3. Lasagna, L. *The Doctors' Dilemmas*. New York: Harper & Brothers, 1962.
4. *New York Times*, January 16, 1991; p. A5.
5. Weinberg, R. J.; Ell, S. R.; Weinberg, E. D. "Blood-Letting, Iron Homeostasis, and Human Health." *Medical Hypotheses*, 1986, 21, 441–443.
6. Weintraub, L. R. "Current Uses of Phlebotomy Therapy." *Hospital Practice* 1987, 22, 251–256 (June 15).
7. Skikne, B.; Lynch, S.; Borek, D.; Cook, J. "Iron and Blood Donation." *Clinics in Haematology* 1984, 13, 271–287.
8. Sullivan, J. L. "Iron and the Sex Difference in Heart Disease Risk." *Lancet* 1981, 1, 1293–1294.
9. Casale, G.; Bignamini, M.; de Nicola, P. "Does Blood Donation Prolong Life Expectancy?" *Vox Sanguinis* 1983, 45, 398–399.
10. Sullivan, J. L. "Is Blood Donation Good For the Donor? Iron, Heart Disease, and Donor Recruitment." *Transfusion*, in press.
11. Surgernor, D. M.; Wallace, E. L.; Hao, S. H. S.; Chapman, R. H. "Collection and Transfusion of Blood in the United States, 1982–1988." *New England Journal of Medicine* 1990, 322, 1646–1651.
12. Altman, L. K. "Europe Supplying Blood for the U.S." *New York Times*, September 5, 1989.
13. Bosy, L. "Donor Recruiters Use Marketing Tactics." *American Medical News* 1987 (Feb. 20), p. 17.
14. Gaul, G. M. "How Blood, the 'Gift of Life,' Became a Billion-

Dollar Business." *Philadelphia Inquirer*, September 21, 1989.

15. Titmuss, R. M. *The Gift Relationship: From Human Blood to Social Policy*. New York: Vantage Press, 1971.

16. American Red Cross. "Blood Donor Information." Form No. 05-007B, Rev. 12/88-100M.

17. Pindyck, J.; Avorn, J.; Kuriyan, M. et al. "Blood Donation by the Elderly: Clinical and Policy Considerations." *Journal of the American Medical Association* 1987, 257, 1186–1188.

18. Huestis, D. W. *Practical Blood Transfusion* (Fourth Edition). Boston: Little, Brown, 1988.

19. Zillmer, E. A.; Glidden, R. A.; Honaker, L. M.; Meyer, J. D. "Mood States in the Volunteer Blood Donor." *Transfusion* 1989, 29, 27–30.

20. Fincher, J. "A Simple Gift of Blood." *Reader's Digest*, October 1988, p. 99.

Chapter 19. One More Reason to Exercise

1. Blair, S. N., Kohl, H.W. III, Paffenbarger, R.S., Clark, D.G., Cooper, K.H., Gibbons, L.W. "Physical Fitness and All-Cause Mortality: A Prospective Study of Healthy Men and Women. *JAMA* 1989; 262: 2395–2401.

2. Ekelund, L.G., Haskell, W.L., Johnson, J.L., Whaley, F.S., Criqui, M.H., Sheps, D.S. "Physical Fitness as a Predictor of Cardiovascular Mortality in Asymptomatic North American Men." The Lipid Research Clinics Mortality Follow-up Study. *New England Journal of Medicine*, 1988; 319: 1379–1384.

3. Vena, J.E., Graham, S., Zielezny, M., Swanson, M.K., Barnes, R.E., Nolan, J. "Lifetime Occupational Exercise and Colon Cancer." *American Journal of Epidemiology*, 1985; 122: 357–65.

4. Simon, H.B. "The Immunology of Exercise. A Brief Review." *Journal of the American Medical Association* 1984; 252: 2735–38.

5. Keast, D., Cameron, K., Morton, A.R. "Exercise and the Immune Response." *Sports Medicine* 1988; 5: 248–67.

6. Lauffer, R. B. "Exercise as Prevention: Do the Health Benefits Derive In Part From Lower Iron Levels?" *Medical Hypotheses* 1991, 35, 103–107.

7. Lauffer, R. B. "Exercise, Fitness and Mortality." *Journal of the American Medical Society* 1990, 263, 2047.

8. Lauffer, R. B. "Iron Depletion and Coronary Disease." *American Heart Journal* 1990, 119, 1448.

9. Saltman, P.; Gurin, J.; Mothner, I. *The California Nutrition Book,* Boston: Little, Brown, 1987.

10. Newhouse, I.J.; Clement, D.B. "Iron Status in Athletes. An Update." *Sports Medicine* 1988; 5: 337–352.

11. Haymes, E. M.; Lamanca, J. J. "Iron Loss in Runners During Exercise: Implications and Recommendations." *Sports Medicine* 1989, 7, 277–285.

12. Blum, S.M., Sherman, A.R., Boileau, R.A. "The Effects of Fitness-Type Exercise on Iron Status in Adult Women." *American Journal of Clinical Nutrition,* 1986; 43: 456–463.

13. Cannon, J.G.; Kluger, M.I. "Endogenous Pyrogen Activity in Human Plasma After Exercise." *Science* (Wash. D.C.) 1983; 220: 617–619.

14. Strachan, A.F., Noakes, T.D., Kotzenberg, G., Nel, A.E., DeBeer, F.C. "C-Reactive Protein Concentrations During Long Distance Running." *British Medical Journal,* 1984; 209. 1249–1251.

15. Campbell, C.H., Solgonick, R.M., Linder, M. "Translational Regulation of Ferritin Synthesis in Rat Spleen: Effects of Iron and Inflammation." *Biochem Biophys Res Commun* 1989; 160: 453–459.

16. Konijn, A.M., Hershko, C. "Ferritin Synthesis in Inflammation. Pathogenesis of Impaired Iron Release." *British Journal of Haematology,* 1977; 37: 7–15.

17. Rogers, J.T.; Bridges, K.R., Durmowicz, G.P., Glass, J., Auron, P.E., Munro, H.N. "Translational Control During the Acute Phase Response. Ferritin Synthesis in Response to Interleukin-1." *Journal of Biological Chemistry* 1990, 265, 14572–14578.

18. Taylor, C., Rogers, G., Goodman, C., Baynes, R.D., Bothwell, T.H., Bezwoda, W.R., Kramer, F., Hattingh, J. "Hematologic, Iron-Related, and Acute-Phase Protein Responses to Sustained Strenuous Exercise." *Journal of Applied Physiology,* 1987; 62: 464–9.

19. Torti, S.V., Kwak, E.L., Miller, S.C., Miller, L.L., Ringold,

G. M., Myambo, K.B., Young, A.P., Torti, F.M., "The Molecular Cloning and Characterization of Murine Ferritin Heavy Chain, a Tumor Necrosis Factor-Inducible Gene." *Journal of Biological Chemistry*, 1988; 263: 12638–12644.

20. Ornish, D. *Dr. Dean Ornish's Program for Reversing Heart Disease.* New York: Random House, 1990.

Glossary

Anemia. Anemia means literally "lack of blood." In medicine, anemia refers to a low concentration of red blood cells or their important contents, hemoglobin, the vital oxygen-carrying substance that contains iron. This causes the patient to feel weary and inefficient, to appear pale, and possibly to experience headaches, slight fever, and physical weakness. Anemia can be caused by abnormal bleeding, excessive destruction of red blood cells, iron or vitamin deficiencies, and other causes. When anemia is caused by iron deficiency, the patient should also have low serum ferritin (less than 12 units) or transferrin saturation (less than 16 percent) readings from blood tests to justify treatment with iron supplements. In addition, the ultimate cause of the anemia, whether related to iron status or not, should always be fully investigated.

Ferritin. Ferritin is a molecular "storage bin" for iron; each ferritin molecule usually contains up to 2000 atoms of iron. It is a protein manufactured by most cells in response to increases in iron availability. It is found both inside cells and in the blood.

Hematocrit. Blood contains cells and a protein-rich liquid called plasma. The percentage of the volume occupied by cells is known as the hematocrit. Normal values are 42 percent for men and 38 percent for women. Since 99 percent of blood cells are red blood cells, the hematocrit is a good indicator of anemia.

Hemochromatosis. Primary, or idiopathic, hemochromatosis is the hereditary iron-overload disease discussed in Chapter 7. Patients with the full-blown form of the disease absorb far greater quantities of iron from their diet than they actually need, resulting in iron accumulation in several organ systems. *Secondary* hemochromatosis refers to iron overload from other causes, such as other genetic diseases, excessive dietary intake of iron, liver disease, blood transfusions.

Hemoglobin. Hemoglobin is the iron-containing, oxygen-carrying substance in red blood cells that gives the cells their color. A

276

low content of hemoglobin in the blood (for example, less than 12 grams per deciliter) indicates anemia but does *not* necessarily mean that the patient is iron)deficient. Normal values for hemoglobin are 14–16.5 grams per deciliter for men and 12–15 grams for women.

Iron stores. See Storage iron

Phlebotomy. Phlebotomy is simply bloodletting through a vein; an equivalent term is *venesection*. It can refer to the removal of any quantity of blood, from small test samples to the pints removed in blood donation and in the treatment of iron overload.

Phytic acid, or phytate. Phytic acid is a phosphorus-rich substance found predominantly in whole grains, legumes, nuts, and seeds. Its ability to bind iron atoms in the intestines reduces iron absorption from the diet and may also protect the intestinal cells from dangerous chemical reactions that are catalyzed by iron.

Red blood cells. Ninety-nine percent of blood cells are red blood cells. These contain hemoglobin, the iron-containing substance that latches on to oxygen in the lungs and carries it to various organs, where it is released.

Serum ferritin. A fraction of the ferritin manufactured in cells to store iron is released into the bloodstream. The level of ferritin in serum, the clear fluid remaining after blood is allowed to clot, is proportional to the total amount of storage iron in the body. Men generally have serum ferritin readings in the range of 30–450 units (nanograms per milliliter or micrograms per liter of serum); premenopausal women, 7–140 units; and older women, 12–170 units. Readings of greater than 300 units suggest iron overload, and readings of less than 12 units are associated with iron deficiency.

Serum iron. While most of the iron in blood is part of the hemoglobin molecule, there is also some iron bound to transferrin, the protein that is free to enter the cells of the body depending on their iron needs. The amount of this form of iron in serum, the clear fluid remaining after blood is allowed to clot, is high in iron overload and low in iron-deficiency anemia. Unfortunately, however, the results of this widely used blood test vary according to the time of day the sample is taken and whether or not the patient has just eaten; thus, it alone is not a good indicator of iron status. (*See also* Transferrin saturation.)

Storage iron. In addition to about 2000 milligrams of iron in hemoglobin and smaller amounts in other important proteins, the body has a reserve of iron stored away in ferritin molecules and *hemosiderin,* a degraded form of ferritin. The amount of this form of iron varies tremendously among different people, from 100–400 milligrams in premenopausal women to values greater than 2000 milligrams for many men and older women. The storage iron itself is not necessarily dangerous; however, the iron can escape from its "storage bins," and it is this form of iron, "free" iron, that *is* dangerous. The total amount of storage iron, in milligrams, can be estimated by multiplying a serum ferritin reading by ten.

Total iron-binding capacity, or TIBC. This is an estimate of the amount of iron that transferrin can bind in blood. It is thus a crude estimate of transferrin content, expressed in units of micrograms of iron that can be bound to 1 deciliter of serum. Normally, both men and women have TIBCs of around 300–360 micrograms of iron per deciliter. Readings less than 300 suggest iron overload, and readings greater than 360 suggest iron deficiency.

Transferrin. Transferrin is the molecular "wheelbarrow" protein, each molecule of which transports up to two atoms of iron in the blood.

Transferrin saturation. The percentage of the iron-binding capacity of blood transferrin that is already filled with iron is known as transferrin saturation. It can be calculated by dividing the result of a serum iron test by the TIBC result and multiplying by 100. Men generally have readings in the range of 10–45 percent, premenopausal women, 10–38 percent, and older women, 17–42 percent. Readings of greater than 62 percent for men and 50 percent for women suggest iron overload, and readings of less than 16 percent are associated with iron deficiency.

Appendix A

Recommended Dietary Allowance (RDA) for Iron[a]

	Group/Age (years)	milligrams of iron
Infants		
	up to six months	6
	six months to one year	10
Children		
	1 to 3	10
	4 to 6	10
	7 to 10	10
Males		
	11 to 14	12
	15 to 18	12
	19 to 24	10
	25 to 50	10
	over 51	10
Females		
	11 to 14	15
	15 to 18	15
	19 to 24	15
	25 to 50	15
	over 51	10
	During pregnancy[b]	15 from diet *plus* 30 from supplement
	Lactating (nursing)[c]	15

ªSources: 1. Committee on Dietary Allowances. "Recommended Dietary Allowances." 10th ed. Washington, D.C.: National Academy of Sciences, 1989.
2. Herbert, V. "Recommended Dietary Intakes (RDI) of Iron in Humans." *American Journal of Clinical Nutrition* 45 (1987): 679–686.

Note: The U.S. RDA for iron, used for nutrition labeling purposes, is currently 18 milligrams. This was the RDA for premenopausal women prior to the 1989 revisions. The U.S. Food and Drug Administration is currently revising the nutritional labeling laws. In 1992, the term Reference Daily Intake, or RDI, will replace Recommended Daily Allowance, and the value for iron will be updated to 15 milligrams.

ᵇThe increased requirement for iron cannot be met by the iron content of the habitual American diet nor by the existing iron stores of many women; therefore, the use of supplements containing 30 milligrams of iron is recommended.

ᶜThe iron needs of lactating women are not substantially different from those of women who are not pregnant, but continued supplementation of the mother for two to three months after giving birth has been recommended to replenish iron stores depleted by pregnancy.

Appendix B

Iron, Vitamin-C, Fat, and Cholesterol Content of Common Foods[a]

Food and Serving Size	Iron (mg.)	Vita-min C (mg.)	Fat (g.)	Choles-terol (mg.)
Beverages				
Beer, 12 fl. oz.	0.11	0	0	0
Coffee, brewed, 6 fl. oz.	0.72	0	0	0
Cola, 12 fl. oz.	0.13	0	0.1	0
Lemonade, from frozen concentrate, 6 fl. oz.	0.41	10	0.1	0
Lemon-lime soda, 12 fl. oz.	0.25	0	0	0
Milk, low-fat, 1% butterfat, 8 fl. oz.	0.12	2	2.6	10
Milk, nonfat, 8 fl. oz.	0.10	2	0.4	4
Milk, whole, 3.7% butterfat, 8 fl. oz.	0.12	4	8.9	35
Tea, black, brewed 3 min, 6 fl. oz.	0.04	0	0	0
Water (tap water), 8 fl. oz.	0.01	0	0	0

[a]Source: Pennington, J. A. T. *Food Values of Portions Commonly Used.* 15th ed. New York: Harper & Row. 1989.

Abbreviations: mg. = milligram; g. = gram; fl. = fluid; oz. = ounce; "—" = not available.

Food and Serving Size	Iron (mg.)	Vita-min C (mg.)	Fat (g.)	Choles-terol (mg.)
Wine, red table wine, 3.5 fl. oz.	0.44	0	0	0
Wine, white table wine, 3.5 fl. oz.	0.33	0	0	0

Candy

Almond Joy, Peter Paul, 1 oz.	0.44	0	2.3	1
Baby Ruth, 2-oz. bar	—	—	12	—
Caramels, 1 oz.	0.4	0	2.9	—
Chocolate, bittersweet, 1 oz.	1.4	0	11.3	—
Chocolate, semisweet, Bakers, ¼ cup	1.11	0	11.8	0
Milk chocolate, 1 oz.	0.3	0	9.2	—
Peanut butter cups, Reese's, 2 pieces (1.8 oz.)	0.56	—	16.7	—

Cereals, Hot

Cream of wheat, instant, cooked, ¾ cup	9.00	—	0.4	—
Oatmeal, instant, Quaker, cooked, ¾ cup	8.1	—	1.7	—

Cereals, Ready-to-eat

Bran, Kellogg's All-Bran, ⅓ cup	4.5	15	0.5	—
Bran flakes, Kellogg's, ¾ cup	8.1	—	0.5	—
Cheerios, General Mills, 1¼ cups	4.45	15	1.8	—

Food and Serving Size	Iron (mg.)	Vita-min C (mg.)	Fat (g.)	Choles-terol (mg.)
Corn Chex, Ralston Purina, 1 cup	1.8	15	0.2	—
Cornflakes, Kellogg's, 1¼ cups	1.8	15	0.1	—
Cracklin' bran, Kellogg's, ⅓ cup	1.8	15	4.1	—
Fruit & fiber, Post, with dates, raisins, walnuts, ½ cup	4.44	0	0.8	0
Granola, Nature Valley, ⅓ cup	0.95	—	4.9	0
Granola, Post Hearty Granola, ¼ cup	4.44	0	4.1	0
Grape-Nuts, Post, ¼ cup	2.67	0	0.1	0
Life, Quaker, ⅔ cup	8.1	—	1.8	—
Nabisco 100% Bran, ⅓ cup	2.7	27.0	1.0	0
Nutri-grain, Kellogg's, wheat, ¾ cup	0.8	15	0.3	—
Oatbake, Kellogg's, ½ cup	4.5	15	3.0	0
Product 19, Kellogg's, ¾ cup	18.0	60	0.2	—
Quaker 100% Natural, ¼ cup	0.85	—	5.6	—
Raisin bran, Kellogg's, ¾ cup	4.5	—	0.7	—
Rice Krispies, Kellogg's, 1 cup	1.8	15	0.2	—
Shredded wheat, 1 oz.	1.2	—	0.6	—

Food and Serving Size	Iron (mg.)	Vita-min C (mg.)	Fat (g.)	Choles-terol (mg.)
Special K, Kellogg's, 1⅓ cups	4.5	15	0.1	—
Total, General Mills, 1 cup	18.0	60	0.6	—
Wheaties, General Mills, 1 cup	4.45	15	0.5	—

Cheese and Cheese Products

Cheddar, 1 oz.	0.19	0	9.4	30
Cottage cheese, low-fat, 2% butterfat, 1 cup	0.36	0	4.4	19
Swiss, 1 oz.	0.05	0	7.1	15

Desserts

Brownie, with nuts, homemade, 1 piece	0.4	0	6.3	—
Cake, angel food, homemade, 1 piece	0.51	0	0.1	—
Cake, carrot, from mix, Duncan Hines Deluxe, 1/12 cake	0.62	—	4.0	0
Cake, cheesecake, 1 piece	0.41	4	16.3	—
Cake, devil's food, from mix, 1/12 cake	0.70	0	11.3	—
Cake, gingerbread, from mix, 1/9 cake	1.0	0	4.3	—
Cake, white, from mix, 1/12 cake	0.50	0	10.2	—
Cookie, chocolate chip, 2	0.38	0	4.4	—

Food and Serving Size	Iron (mg.)	Vita- min C (mg.)	Fat (g.)	Choles- terol (mg.)
Cookie, oatmeal raisin, 4	1.5	0	8.0	—
Cookie, sugar, homemade, 2	0.22	0	2.7	—
Danish pastry, 1 piece	0.78	0	8.8	—
Doughnut, glazed old-fashioned, Hostess, 1	—	0	12.0	11
Ice cream, vanilla, regular (10% butterfat), 1 cup	0.12	1	14.3	59
Pie, apple, homemade, ⅛ pie	1.06	0	11.9	—
Pie, pumpkin, homemade, ⅛ pie	0.60	0	12.8	—
Sherbet, orange, 1 cup	0.31	4	3.8	14
Eggs and Egg Dishes				
Egg, boiled, hard or soft, 1 large	1.04	0	5.6	274
Egg white, fresh or frozen, 1	0.01	0	0	0
Egg yolk, fresh, 1	0.95	0	5.6	272
Quiche, bacon and onion, Pour-a-Quiche, 4.3 oz.	—	—	18.0	240
Fast Foods				
Burger King chicken sandwich	3.3	—	40.0	82
Burger King hamburger	2.73	3	12.0	37

Food and Serving Size	Iron (mg.)	Vita-min C (mg.)	Fat (g.)	Choles-terol (mg.)
Burger King Whaler sandwich	2.22	—	27.0	84
Burger King Whopper	4.88	14	41.0	94
Kentucky Fried Chicken, original recipe, breast	0.63	—	13.7	93
Kentucky Fried Chicken, original recipe, drumstick	0.60	—	8.8	81
McDonald's Big Mac	4.9	3	35.0	83
McDonald's Chicken McNuggets, 1 serving	1.25	2	21.3	73
McDonald's Egg McMuffin	2.93	—	15.8	259
McDonald's Filet-o-Fish sandwich	2.47	—	25.7	45
McDonald's french fries, 1 regular serving	0.61	13	11.5	9
McDonald's hamburger	2.85	2	11.3	29
McDonald's McDLT	6.60	8	44.0	101
McDonald's Quarter Pounder	4.30	3	23.5	81
Pizza, cheese, 1 slice	1.61	2	8.6	56
Taco, 1	1.15	1	10.4	21

Food and Serving Size	Iron (mg.)	Vita-min C (mg.)	Fat (g.)	Choles-terol (mg.)
Fish, Shellfish, and Crustacea				
Clams, raw, 3 oz. (4 large or 9 small)	11.88	—	0.8	29
Cod, baked or broiled, 3 oz.	0.41	1	0.7	47
Crab, Alaska king, raw, 3 oz.	0.5	—	0.5	35
Fish sticks, frozen, 1 stick	0.21	—	3.4	31
Haddock, baked or broiled, 3 oz.	1.14	—	0.8	63
Halibut, baked or broiled, 3 oz.	0.91	—	2.5	35
Lobster, boiled, 3 oz.	0.33	—	0.5	61
Oysters, raw, 6 medium	5.63	—	2.1	46
Salmon, pink, canned with bone, 3 oz.	0.72	0	5.1	—
Scallops, raw, 3 oz. (6 large or 14 small)	0.25	—	0.6	28
Shrimp, boiled, 3 oz. (15 large)	2.62	—	0.9	166
Swordfish, baked or broiled, 3 oz.	0.88	1	4.4	43
Tuna, canned in oil, light, 3 oz.	1.18	—	7.0	15
Tuna, canned in oil, white, 3 oz.	0.56	—	6.9	26
Tuna, canned in spring water, light, 3 oz.	2.72	—	0.4	—

Food and Serving Size	Iron (mg.)	Vita- min C (mg.)	Fat (g.)	Choles- terol (mg.)
Tuna, canned in spring water, white, 3 oz.	0.51	—	2.1	35

Fruit and Vegetable Juices

Apple juice, canned or bottled, 8 fl. oz.	0.92	2	0.3	0
Grapefruit juice, canned, 8 fl. oz.	0.50	72	0.2	0
Orange juice, from frozen concentrate, 8 fl. oz.	0.24	97	0.1	0
Tomato juice, 6 fl. oz.	1.06	33	0.1	0
V-8 vegetable cocktail, Campbell's, 6 fl. oz.	1.00	37	0.1	—

Fruits

Apple, with skin, 1 medium	0.25	8	0.5	0
Cantaloupe, pieces, 1 cup	0.34	68	0.4	0
Grapefuit, pink or red, ½ medium	0.15	47	0.1	0
Grapes, American (slip skin), 1 cup	0.27	4	0.3	0
Honeydew melon, pieces, ¼ cup	0.40	23	0.3	—
Orange, navel, 1 medium	0.17	80	0.1	0
Peach, fresh, 1 medium	0.10	6	0.1	0

Food and Serving Size	Iron (mg.)	Vita-min C (mg.)	Fat (g.)	Choles-terol (mg.)
Pear, fresh, 1 medium	0.41	7	0.7	0
Pineapple, canned, in heavy syrup, 1 cup	0.98	19	0.3	0
Prunes, dried, 10 prunes	2.08	3	0.4	0
Raisins, seedless, ⅔ cup	2.08	3	0.5	0
Strawberries, fresh, 1 cup	0.57	85	0.6	0
Watermelon, pieces, 1 cup	0.28	15	0.7	0
Grain Products				
Bagel	1.46	0	1.4	—
Corn bread, from mix, 1 piece	0.80	0	5.8	—
French bread, 1 slice	0.92	—	1.1	—
Pita bread, 1 "pocket"	0.92	0	0.6	—
Pumpernickel bread, 1 slice	0.88	0	0.8	—
Raisin bread, 1 slice	0.78	0	1.0	—
Rye bread, 1 slice	0.68	0	0.9	—
Spaghetti, enriched, cooked, 1 cup	2.25	0	0.7	0
White bread, 1 slice	0.68	0	0.9	—
Whole wheat bread, 1 slice	0.84	0	1.0	—

Food and Serving Size	Iron (mg.)	Vita- min C (mg.)	Fat (g.)	Choles- terol (mg.)
Meats and Poultry				
Beef, corned, cured brisket, cooked, 3.5 oz.	1.86	16	19.0	98
Beef, ground, extra lean, pan-fried, 3.5 oz.	2.36	0	16.4	91
Beef, frankfurter, 1	0.81	14	16.3	35
Beef, ground, regular, pan-fried	2.45	0	22.6	89
Beef, liver, pan-fried, 3.5 oz.	6.28	23	8.0	482
Beef, round, top, separable lean and fat, broiled, 3.5 oz.	2.81	0	8.8	85
Beef, short-loin T-bone steak, lean and fat, broiled, 3.5 oz. separable	2.54	0	24.6	84
Chicken, dark meat without skin, roast, 3.5 oz.	1.33	0	9.7	93
Chicken, light meat without skin, roast, 3.5 oz.	1.14	0	10.9	84
Lamb, leg, roast, 3 oz.	1.40	—	16.1	—
Pork, center loin, pan-fried, 3.5 oz.	0.84	0	30.5	103
Pork, cured bacon, broiled or pan-fried, 3 medium pieces	0.31	6	9.4	16

Food and Serving Size	Iron (mg.)	Vita-min C (mg.)	Fat (g.)	Choles-terol (mg.)
Pork, cured ham, regular, canned, 3.5 oz.	0.83	22	13.0	39
Turkey, dark meat without skin, roast, 3.5 oz.	2.33	0	7.2	85
Turkey, light meat without skin, roast, 3.5 oz.	1.35	0	3.2	69
Nuts and Seeds				
Almonds, toasted, 1 oz.	1.40	0	14.4	0
Cashews, dry-roasted, 1 oz.	1.70	0	13.2	0
Coconut, dried, sweetened, 1 cup	1.33	0	23.8	0
Peanut butter, Skippy, 1 tablespoon	0.30	0	8.2	0
Peanuts, dry-roasted, 1 oz.	0.63	0	13.9	0
Sunflower seeds, dry-roasted, 1 oz.	1.1	0	14.1	0
Walnuts, black, dried, 1 oz.	0.87	—	16.1	0
Vegetables				
Asparagus, boiled, 6 spears	0.59	18	0.3	0
Avocado, raw, California, 1 medium	2.04	14	30.0	0
Beans, baked, Campbell's, 7.9 oz.	3.00	5	4.0	—

Food and Serving Size	Iron (mg.)	Vita-min C (mg.)	Fat (g.)	Choles-terol (mg.)
Broccoli, boiled, ½ cup	0.89	49	0.2	0
Cabbage, green, boiled, ½ cup	0.29	18	0.1	0
Carrot, raw, 1 medium	0.36	7	0.1	0
Cauliflower, boiled, ½ cup	0.26	34	0.1	0
Celery, raw, 1 stalk	0.19	3	0.1	0
Chickpeas (garbanzo beans), canned, 1 cup	3.23	9	2.7	0
Corn, yellow, boiled, ½ cup	0.50	5	1.1	0
Green beans (snap beans), boiled, ½ cup	0.79	6	0.2	0
Kidney beans, red, boiled, 1 cup	5.20	2	0.9	0
Lettuce, iceberg, 1 leaf	0.1	1	0.0	0
Lima beans, boiled, 1 cup	4.36	0	0.7	0
Mushrooms, raw, ½ cup sliced	0.43	1	0.2	0
Onions, boiled, ½ cup	0.21	6	0.2	0
Peas, green, boiled, ½ cup	1.24	11	0.2	0
Peppers, sweet, raw, ½ cup	0.63	64	0.2	0
Potato, baked with skin, 1	2.75	26	0.2	0
Rice, brown, cooked, 1 cup	1.00	0	1.2	

Food and Serving Size	Iron (mg.)	Vita-min C (mg.)	Fat (g.)	Choles-terol (mg.)
Rice, white, enriched, cooked, 1 cup	1.80	0	0.2	0
Spinach, boiled, ½ cup	3.21	9	0.1	0
Sweet potato, baked, 1	0.52	28	0.1	0
Tomato, red, raw, 1 medium	0.59	22	0.3	0

Appendix C

Iron and Vitamin-C Content of Selected Supplements[a]

Product Name	Company Name	Iron Content milligrams	Iron Content % RDA[b]	Vitamin-C Content milligrams	Vitamin-C Content % RDA
A. C. N. tablets	Person & Covey	—	—	250	417%
Albee C-800 tablets	Robins	—	—	800	1333%
Albee C-800 Plus Iron tablets	Robins	27	150%	800	1333%
Albee-T tablets	Robins	—	—	500	833%
Arbon	Forest	18	100%	60	100%
Avail tablets	Beecham	18	100%	90	150%
B.C.E. & Zinc tablets	Schein	—	—	600	1000%
Becotin with C pulvules	Dista	—	—	150	250%
Bee-T-Vites tablets	Rugby	—	—	300	500%

[a]Source: American Pharmaceutical Association. *Handbook of Nonprescription Drugs.* 9th ed. Washington, D.C., 1990.
[b]Based on the current U.S. RDA for iron of 18 milligrams.
[c]Based on the current U.S. RDA for vitamin C of 60 milligrams.

Product Name	Company Name	Iron Content milligrams	% RDA[b]	Vitamin-C Content milligrams	% RDA
Bee-Zee tablets	Rugby	—	—	600	1000%
Beminal-500 tablets	Whitehall	—	—	500	833%
Beminal Stress Plus with Iron tablets	Whitehall	27	150%	700	1167%
Beminal Stress Plus with Zinc tablets	Whitehall	—	—	700	1167%
Bugs Bunny children's chewable tablets	Miles	—	—	60	100%
Bugs Bunny Plus Iron chewable tablets	Miles	15	83%	60	100%
Bugs Bunny Vitamins & Minerals chewable tablets	Miles	18	100%	60	100%
Bugs Bunny with Extra C children's chewable tablets	Miles	—	—	250	417%
C & E capsules	Nature's Bounty	—	—	500	833%
Cal-Prenal Improved tablets	Vortech	49.3	274%	50	83%
Centrovite Jr. tablets	Rugby	18	100%	60	100%
Centrum	Lederle	18	100%	60	100%

Product Name	Company Name	Iron Content		Vitamin-C Content	
		milligrams	% RDA[b]	milligrams	% RDA
Centrum Jr. Plus Iron tablets	Lederle	18	100%	60	100%
Chel-Iron liquid	Kinney	50 (5 milliliters)	278%	—	—
Chel-Iron pediatric drops	Kinney	25 (1 milliliter)	139%	—	—
Chel-Iron tablets	Kinney	40	222%	—	—
Chew-Vites chewable tablets	Vortech	—	—	60	100%
Clusivol syrup	Whitehall	(5 milliliters)	—	15	25%
Daily-Vite with Iron & Minerals tablets	Rugby	18	100%	60	100%
Dayalets filmtabs	Abbott	—	—	60	100%
Daylets Plus Iron filmtabs	Abbott	18	100%	60	100%
Decagen Tabs	Goldline	30	167%	90	150%
Ecee Plus tablets	Edwards	—	—	100	167%
Econo B & C caplets	Vangard	—	—	300	500%
En-Cebrin Pulvules	Lilly	30	167%	50	83%
Engram-HP tablets	Squibb	9	50%	30	50%
Femiron	SmithKline Beecham	20	111%	—	—

Product Name	Company Name	Iron Content milligrams	% RDA[b]	Vitamin-C Content milligrams	% RDA
Femiron tablets	Beecham	20	111%	60	100%
Feosol capsules	SmithKline	50	278%	—	—
Feosol tablets	SmithKline	65	361%	—	—
Feosol elixir	SmithKline	44	244%	—	—
		(5 milliliters)			
Feostat chewable tablets	Forest	33	183%	—	—
Feostat drops	Forest	15	83%	—	—
		(0.6 milliliter)			
Feostat suspension	Forest	33	183%	—	—
		(5 milliliters)			
Ferancee	Stuart	67	372%	150	250%
Ferancee-HP	Stuart	110	611%	600	1000%
Fergon elixir	Winthrop	35	194%	—	—
		(5 milliliters)			
Fergon tablets	Winthrop	37	206%	—	—
Fergon Plus caplets	Winthrop	58	322%	75	125%
Fer-In-Sol capsules	Mead Johnson	60	333%	—	—
Fer-In-Sol drops	Mead Johnson	15	83%	—	—
		(0.6 milliliter)			
Fer-In-Sol syrup	Mead Johnson	18	100%	—	—
		(5 milliliters)			
Fermalox tablets	Rorer	40	222%	—	—

Product Name	Company Name	Iron Content milligrams	% RDA[b]	Vitamin-C Content milligrams	% RDA
Fero-Grad-500 tablets	Abbott	105	583%	500	833%
Fero-Gradumet tablets	Abbott	105	583%	—	—
Ferralyn lanacaps	Lannett	50	278%	—	—
Ferra-TD capsules	Goldline	50	278%	—	—
Ferro-Dok TR capsules	Major	50	278%	—	—
Ferro-Sequels	Lederle	50	278%	—	—
Ferrous-S.Q.L. capsules	Goldline	50	278%	—	—
Filibon tablets	Lederle	18	100%	60	100%
Flintstones children's chewable tablets	Miles	—	—	60	100%
Flintstones Complete chewable tablets	Miles	18	100%	60	100%
Flintstones Plus Iron chewable tablets	Miles	15	83%	60	100%
Flintstones with Extra C children's chewable tablets	Miles	—	—	250	417%
Fruity Chews chewable tablets	Goldline	—	—	60	100%
Fruity Chews with Iron chewable tablets	Goldline	12	67%	60	100%
Fumaral Elixir	Vortech	45	250%	200	333%

Product Name	Company Name	Iron Content		Vitamin-C Content	
		milligrams	% RDA[b]	milligrams	% RDA
Fumaral spancaps	Vortech	108	600%	200	333%
Gen-bee with C caplets	Goldline	—	—	300	500%
Generet-500 tablets	Goldline	105	583%	500	833%
Generix-T tablets	Goldline	15	83%	150	250%
Geriamic tablets	Vortech	50	278%	75	125%
Geriot tablets	Goldline	50	278%	75	125%
Geriplex-FS kapseals	Parke-Davis	6	33%	50	83%
Geriplex-FS liquid	Parke-Davis	2.5 (5 milliliters)	14%	—	—
Geritol Complete tablets	SmithKline Beecham	50	278%	60	100%
Geritol Extend	SmithKline Beecham	10	56%	60	100%
Geritol liquid	SmithKline Beecham	50 (15 milliliters)	277%	—	—
Gevrabon liquid	Lederle	2.5 (5 milliliters)	14%	—	—
Gevral Protein	Lederle	4.3	24%	22	37%
Gevral T tablets	Lederle	27	150%	90	150%
Gevral tablets	Lederle	18	100%	60	100%
Gevrite	Lederle	18	100%	60	100%
Hep-Forte capsules	Marlyn	—	—	10	17%

Product Name	Company Name	Iron Content		Vitamin-C Content	
		milligrams	% RDA[b]	milligrams	% RDA
Hepicebrin tablets	Lilly	—	—	75	125%
Herbal Cellulex tablets	Nature's Bounty	9	50%	83	138%
Homicebrin liquid	Lilly	—	—	60	100%
		(5 milliliters)			
Hytinic capsules	Hyrex	150	833%	—	—
Hytinic elixir	Hyrex	20	111%	—	—
		(1 milliliter)			
Iberet filmtabs	Abbott	105	583%	150	250%
Iberet-500 filmtabs	Abbott	105	583%	500	833%
Iberet-Liquid	Abbott	78.75	438%	375	642%
		(15 milliliters)			
Iberet-500 Liquid	Abbott	78.75	438%	112.5	188%
		(15 milliliters)			
Iberol filmtabs	Abbott	105	583%	75	125%
Ibex therapeutic tablets	Freeda	16.5	92%	150	250%
Incremin with Iron syrup	Lederle	90	500%	—	—
		(15 milliliters)			
KLB6 Complete tablets	Nature's Bounty	—	—	10	17%
Livitamin capsules	Beecham Labs	33	183%	100	167%
Livitamin chewables	Beecham Labs	16.5	92%	100	167%
Livitamin liquid	Beecham Labs	35.5	197%	75	125%
		(15 milliliters)			

Product Name	Company Name	Iron Content milligrams	% RDA[b]	Vitamin-C Content milligrams	% RDA
Mediplex Tabules tablets	US Pharm	—	—	300	500%
Mi-Cebrin tablets	Dista	15	83%	100	167%
Mi-Cebrin T tablets	Dista	15	83%	150	250%
Mol-Iron tablets	Schering	39	217%	—	—
Mol-Iron with Vitamin C	Schering	39	217%	75	125%
Multi Vit drops	Barre-National	— (1 milliliter)	—	35	58%
Multicebrin tablets	Lilly	—	—	75	125%
Multilex tablets	Rugby	15	83%	100	167%
Multilex-T & M tablets	Rugby	15	83%	150	250%
Multi-Mineral tablets	Nature's Bounty	3	17%	—	—
Multi-Vita-Drops	PBI	—	—	35	58%
Multi-Vita Drops with Iron	PBI	10 (1 milliliter)	56%	35	58%
Myadec tablets	Parke-Davis	30	167%	90	150%
Natabec kapseals	Parke-Davis	30	167%	50	83%
Natabec FA capsules	Parke-Davis	30	167%	50	83%
Natalins tablets	Mead Johnson	45	250%	90	150%
NeoVadrin Centurion tablets	Scherer	27	150%	90	150%
NeoVadrin children's chewable tablets with iron	Mission	15	83%	60	100%

Product Name	Company Name	Iron Content		Vitamin-C Content	
		milligrams	*% RDA*[b]	*milligrams*	*% RDA*
NeoVadrin prenatal tablets	Mission	60	333%	60	100%
Niferex capsules	Central	150	833%	—	—
Niferex tablets	Central	50	278%	—	—
Niferex elixir	Central	20 (1 milliliter)	111%	—	—
Niferex with Vitamin C tablets	Central	50	278%	100	167%
Norlac tablets	Reid-Rowell	60	333%	90	150%
Nova-Dec tablets	Rugby	20	111%	250	417%
One-A-Day Essential tablets	Miles	—	—	60	100%
One-A-Day Maximum Formula tablets	Miles	18	100%	60	100%
One-A-Day Plus Extra C tablets	Miles	—	—	300	500%
One-A-Day Stressgard tablets	Miles	18	100%	600	1000%
Optilets-500 filmtabs	Abbott	—	—	500	833%
Optilets-M-500 filmtabs	Abbott	20	111%	500	833%
Optivite for Women tablets	Optimox	2.5	14%	250	417%

Product Name	Company Name	Iron Content milligrams	% RDA[b]	Vitamin-C Content milligrams	% RDA
Os-Cal Forte tablets	Marion	5	28%	50	83%
Os-Cal Plus tablets	Marion	16.6	92%	33	55%
Oxi-Freeda tablets	Freeda	—	—	100	167%
Peritinic tablets	Lederle	100	556%	200	333%
Poly-Vi-Sol chewable tablets	Mead Johnson	—	—	60	100%
Poly-Vi-Sol infants' drops	Mead Johnson	— (1 milliliter)	—	35	58%
Poly-Vi-Sol with Iron drops	Mead Johnson	12 (1 milliliter)	67%	60	100%
Polyvitamin Drops with Iron	Rugby	10 (1 milliliter)	56%	35	58%
Prenatal with Folic Acid tablets	Geneva Generics	60	333%	60	100%
Prenatal-S tablets	Goldline	—	—	100	167%
Prenavite tablets	Rugby	60	333%	60	100%
Probec-T tablets	Stuart	—	—	600	1000%
Rogenic tablets	Forest	100	556%	200	333%
Ru-lets 500 tablets	Rugby	—	—	500	833%
Secran/Fe elixir	Scherer	90 (15 milliliters)	500%	—	—
Sigtab tablets	Upjohn	—	—	333	555%
Simron capsules	Lakeside	10	56%	—	—

Product Name	Company Name	Iron Content		Vitamin-C Content	
		milligrams	*% RDA*[b]	*milligrams*	*% RDA*
Simron Plus capsules	Merrell Dow	10	56%	50	83%
Slow Fe tablets	Ciba	50	278%	—	—
Spartus tablets	Lederle	—	—	300	500%
Stress Formula 600 Plus Zinc tablets	Schein	—	—	600	1000%
Stress-Bee capsules	Rugby	—	—	300	500%
Stress capsules	Lederle	—	—	300	500%
Stressgard tablets	Miles	18	100%	600	1000%
Stresstabs 600 Advanced Formula tablets	Lederle	—	—	600	1000%
Stresstabs 600 with Iron tablets	Lederle	27	150%	600	1000%
Stresstabs 600 with Zinc tablets	Lederle	—	—	600	1000%
Stuart Prenatal tablets	Stuart	60	333%	100	167%
Stuart Formula tablets	Stuart	18	100%	60	100%
Stuartinic tablets	Stuart	100	556%	500	833%
Sunkist Multis regular	Ciba	—	—	60	100%
Sunkist Multis Plus C	Ciba	—	—	250	417%
Sunkist Multis Plus Iron	Ciba	15	83%	60	100%
Sunkist Multis Complete	Ciba	18	100%	60	100%

Product Name	Company Name	Iron Content		Vitamin-C Content	
		milligrams	*% RDA*[b]	*milligrams*	*% RDA*
Surbex-750 with Iron filmtabs	Abbott	27	150%	750	1250%
Surbex-750 with Zinc filmtabs	Abbott	—	—	750	1250%
Surbex-T filmtabs	Abbott	—	—	500	833%
Surbex with C filmtabs	Abbott	—	—	250	417%
Surbu-Gen-T tablets	Goldline	—	—	500	833%
Thera Multivitamin liquid	Major	— (5 milliliters)	—	200	333%
Thera-Combex H-P kapseals	Parke-Davis	—	—	500	833%
Theragenerix tablets	Goldline	—	—	120	200%
Theragenerix-M tablets	Goldline	27	150%	120	200%
Theragran Jr. children's chewable tablets	Squibb	—	—	60	100%
Theragran Jr. children's chewable tablets with extra vitamin C	Squibb	—	—	250	417%
Theragran Jr. with Iron chewable tablets	Squibb	18	100%	60	100%

Product Name	Company Name	Iron Content		Vitamin-C Content	
		milligrams	% RDA[b]	milligrams	% RDA
Theragran liquid	Squibb	— (5 milliliters)	—	200	333%
Theragran-M tablets	Squibb	27	150%	120	200%
Theragran Stress Formula tablets	Squibb	27	150%	600	1000%
Theragran tablets	Squibb	—	—	90	150%
Theravee tablets	Vangard	—	—	120	200%
Theravee-M tablets	Vangard	27	150%	120	200%
Therems tablets	Rugby	—	—	120	200%
Therems-M tablets	Rugby	27	150%	120	200%
ThexForte caplets	Medtech	—	—	500	833%
Tri-Vi-Sol drops	Mead Johnson	— (1 milliliter)	—	35	58%
Tri-Vi-Sol with Iron drops	Mead Johnson	10	56%	35	58%
Troph-Iron liquid	SmithKline	20 (1 milliliter)	111%	—	—
Ultra Freeda tablets	Freeda	5 (5 milliliters)	28%	333	555%
Unicap capsules, tablets, and chewable tablets	Upjohn	—	—	60	100%
Unicap M tablets	Upjohn	18	100%	60	100%
Unicap Plus Iron tablets	Upjohn	22.5	125%	60	100%

Product Name	Company Name	Iron Content		Vitamin-C Content	
		milligrams	*% RDA*[b]	*milligrams*	*% RDA*
Unicap Senior tablets	Upjohn	10	56%	60	100%
Unicap T tablets	Upjohn	18	100%	500	833%
Unicomplex M tablets	Rugby	18	100%	60	100%
Unicomplex T&M tablets	Rugby	10	56%	300	500%
Vicon C capsules	Russ	—	—	300	500%
Vicon Plus capsules	Russ	—	—	150	250%
Vi-Daylin ADC Vitamins Plus Iron drops	Ross	10 (1 milliliter)	56%	35	58%
Vi-Daylin chewable tablets	Ross	—	—	60	100%
Vi-Daylin Multivitamin liquid	Ross	—	—	60	100%
Vi-Daylin Multivitamin Plus Iron chewable tablets	Ross	12	67%	60	100%
Vi-Daylin Multivitamin Plus Iron drops	Ross	10 (1 milliliter)	56%	35	58%
Vi-Daylin Plus Iron liquid	Ross	10 (5 milliliters)	56%	60	100%
Vigortol liquid	Rugby	10 (15 milliliters)	56%	—	—
Vigran tablets	Squibb	—	—	60	100%

Product Name	Company Name	Iron Content milligrams	% RDA[b]	Vitamin-C Content milligrams	% RDA
Vio-Bec capsules	Reid-Rowell	—	—	500	833%
Vio-Bec Forte tablets	Reid-Rowell	—	—	500	833%
Viogen-C capsules	Goldline	—	—	300	500%
Vita Bee C-800 tablets	Rugby	—	—	800	1333%
Vita-bee with C captabs	Rugby	—	—	300	500%
Vitagett tablets	Vortech	13.4	74%	50	83%
Vita-Kaps filmtabs	Abbott	—	—	50	83%
Vita-Kaps-M tablets	Abbott	10	56%	50	83%
Vitamin-Mineral-Supplement liquid	PBI	2.5 (5 milliliters)	14%	—	—
Vitron-C	Fisons	66	367%	125	208%
Vitron-C Plus	Fisons	132	733%	250	417%
Vi-Zac capsules	Russ	—	—	500	833%
Within tablets	Miles	27	150%	60	100%
Zentinic pulvule capsules	Lilly	100	556%	200	333%
Zentron liquid	Lilly	60 (15 milliliters)	333%	300	500%
Z-Bec tablets	Robins	—	—	600	1000%
Z-gen tablets	Goldline	—	—	600	1000%
Zymacap capsules	Upjohn	—	—	90	150%

Appendix D

Useful Addresses and Phone Numbers

Please feel free to write the author at the following address:

Dr. Randall B. Lauffer
Massachusetts General Hospital
MRI Center
Building 149, 2nd Floor
13th Street
Charlestown, MA 02129

Other addresses:

American Association of Blood Banks
1117 North 19th Street, Suite 600
Arlington, VA 22209
(703) 528-8200

American Cancer Society, Inc.
1599 Clifton Road NE
Atlanta, GA 30329
(404) 320-3333

American Heart Association National Center
7320 Greenville Avenue
Dallas, TX 75231
(214) 373-6300

American Red Cross National Headquarters
431 18th Street NW
Washington, D.C. 20006
(202) 737-8300

Center for Science In the Public Interest
1501 16th Street NW
Washington, D.C. 20036
(202) 332-9110

Council of Community Blood Centers
1725 15th Street NW, Suite 700
Washington, D.C. 20005
(202) 393-5725

The Hemochromatosis Research Foundation, Inc.
P.O. Box 8569
Albany, NY 12208
(518) 489-0972

Iron Overload Diseases Association
433 Westwind Drive
North Palm Beach, FL 33408
(407) 840-8512

Appendix E

The IRON BALANCE Diary

Date	Blood Donation	Blood Test	Serum Ferritin Result x 10 = (ng/ml or μg/l)	Estimated Iron Stores (mg)	Comments or Other Test Results

About the Author

Randall B. Lauffer holds a Ph.D. in chemistry from Cornell University. Currently an assistant professor at Harvard Medical School, Dr. Lauffer is an expert on mineral biochemistry and the use of minerals in medical diagnosis and therapy. He has published over fifty scientific papers and is currently editing and cowriting a technical book on iron and human health. He lives in Boston, where he directs a research lab at Massachusetts General Hospital. Dr. Lauffer has also founded a pharmaceutical research company, Metasyn, Inc., which is focused on finding new medical applications of mineral biochemistry.

Index